The British Medical Association

FAMILY DOCTOR GUIDE *to*

BLOOD PRESSURE

DK The British ☤ Medical Association

BLOOD PRESSURE

PROFESSOR D.G. BEEVERS

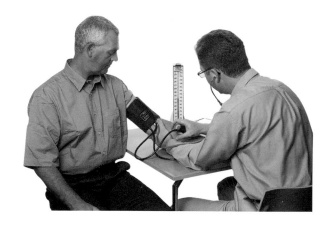

MEDICAL EDITOR
DR. TONY SMITH

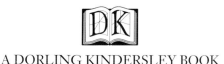

DK

A DORLING KINDERSLEY BOOK

IMPORTANT

This book is intended not as a substitute for personal medical advice but as a supplement to that advice for the patient who wishes to understand more about his/her condition.

Before taking any form of treatment YOU SHOULD ALWAYS CONSULT YOUR MEDICAL PRACTITIONER

In particular (without limit) you should note that advances in medical science occur rapidly and some of the information about drugs and treatment contained in this booklet may very soon be out of date.

PLEASE NOTE
The author regrets that he cannot enter into any correspondence with readers.

DORLING KINDERSLEY
LONDON, NEW YORK, AUCKLAND, DELHI,
JOHANNESBURG, MUNICH, PARIS AND SYDNEY

DK www.dk.com

Senior Editors Nicki Lampon, Mary Lindsay
Senior Designers Jan English, Sarah Hall
Production Controller Elizabeth Cherry

Managing Editor Martyn Page
Managing Art Editor Bryn Walls

Produced for Dorling Kindersley Limited by
Design Revolution, Queens Park Villa,
30 West Drive, Brighton, East Sussex BN2 2GE
Editorial Director Ian Whitelaw
Art Director Becky Willis
Editor Julie Whitaker
Designer Andrew Easton

Published in Great Britain in 2000 by
Dorling Kindersley Limited,
9 Henrietta Street, London WC2E 8PS

2 4 6 8 10 9 7 5 3 1

ISBN 07513 08153

Reproduced by Colourscan, Singapore
Printed in Hong Kong by Wing King Tong

Contents

Introduction

If you are over the age of 30 and cannot remember when you last had your blood pressure checked, you could be one of the 7–10 million people in the UK who has high blood pressure. Doctors usually use the term 'hypertension' to describe this condition, which may cause no symptoms at all for very many years, but could eventually lead to serious complications, including heart disease and strokes.

A COMMON PROBLEM
In the UK, between 10 and 20 per cent of the population suffer from hypertension.

In this book, the word hypertension is used to mean a blood pressure level that has been found on several separate occasions to be above normal and that needs treating to prevent complications developing in the long term.

The condition is very common in the UK, where 10–20 per cent of the population have hypertension, and, the older you are, the more likely you are to have developed it.

Whether you do so depends on a number of related factors, including heredity, your diet – and especially the amounts of salt and alcohol you consume – your ethnic background, whether you have diabetes or you

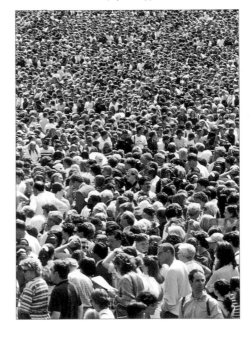

are overweight and whether you take regular exercise.

If all this sounds alarming, there is good news too. Hypertension can be easily diagnosed: your blood pressure can be measured quickly and painlessly at your GP's surgery or health centre. When the reading is above normal, the check can be repeated three or four times if necessary to establish that the first figure was not a chance finding.

Even if you do have hypertension, you may be one of the many people who do not need drug treatment for some time (and possibly not ever), provided you make some straightforward lifestyle changes that will not only lower your blood pressure but bring general health benefits too. When treatment is required, there are a number of very effective drugs available, which are taken in tablet form usually once or twice daily. Most people find that they have no problems at all with the treatment, but, if you do experience side-effects from one drug, there are other, equally effective alternatives. More modern drugs tend to have very few side-effects. Research has shown that controlling hypertension with drug therapy can bring down the risk of a stroke by 35–40 per cent, and the risk of coronary heart disease by 20–25 per cent.

The most important message on hypertension is that, unless you have your blood pressure checked, you may not know that you have hypertension until it has done you serious damage. Even quite seriously raised blood pressure can be controlled once it is identified and, provided that you keep taking the treatment prescribed and have regular check-ups, your chances of developing serious and potentially life-threatening complications are dramatically reduced.

KEY POINTS

- Hypertension affects between seven and ten million people in the UK.

- Hypertension is often not diagnosed.

- The treatment of hypertension saves lives.

What is blood pressure?

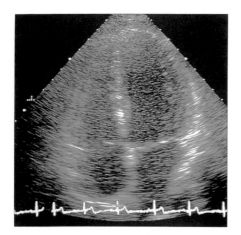

When doctors talk about blood pressure, what they mean is the pressure in the large blood vessels as your heart forces blood around your body. On the whole, the lower your blood pressure, the healthier you are in the long term (except in some very rare conditions in which excessively low blood pressure is part of a disease).

ECHOCARDIOGRAM
This echocardiogram shows the heart. An echocardiogram reveals the size and shape of the heart chambers and valves, the movement of the muscular walls of the heart chamber and the opening and closing of the four valves.

THE CIRCULATORY SYSTEM

Blood picks up oxygen in the lungs from the air that we breathe in. This oxygenated blood enters the heart and is then pumped out to all parts of the body in blood vessels called arteries. Larger blood vessels branch into smaller and smaller ones and then to microscopic arterioles, which eventually form tiny networks of blood vessels known as capillaries. This network of larger arteries, medium-sized arterioles and tiny capillaries allows blood to reach every cell of the body and deposit its oxygen, which is used by cells to make the vital energy they need to survive. Once the blood has

The Sequence that Makes Up a Heartbeat

The heartbeat sequence has three phases – diastole, atrial systole and ventricular systole. The timing of these phases must be accurately maintained, regardless of how slowly or rapidly the heart is beating.

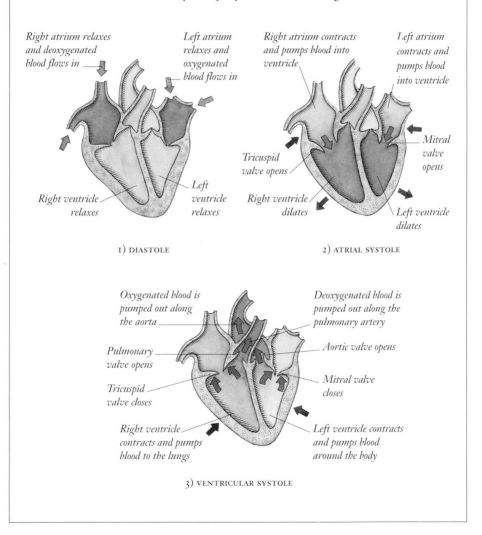

Right atrium relaxes and deoxygenated blood flows in

Left atrium relaxes and oxygenated blood flows in

Right atrium contracts and pumps blood into ventricle

Left atrium contracts and pumps blood into ventricle

Tricuspid valve opens

Mitral valve opens

Right ventricle relaxes

Left ventricle relaxes

Right ventricle dilates

Left ventricle dilates

1) DIASTOLE

2) ATRIAL SYSTOLE

Oxygenated blood is pumped out along the aorta

Deoxygenated blood is pumped out along the pulmonary artery

Pulmonary valve opens

Aortic valve opens

Tricuspid valve closes

Mitral valve closes

Right ventricle contracts and pumps blood to the lungs

Left ventricle contracts and pumps blood around the body

3) VENTRICULAR SYSTOLE

11

deposited its oxygen in the cells, the deoxygenated blood returns to the heart in veins, to be pumped back up to the lungs to pick up more oxygen.

During each heartbeat, the heart muscle contracts to push blood around the body. The pressure produced by the heart is highest when it contracts, and this is known as the systolic (higher value) pressure. Then the heart muscle relaxes before its next contraction, and the pressure is at its lowest, which is known as the diastolic (lower value) pressure. Both systolic and diastolic pressures are measured when you have your blood pressure checked.

The dividing line between a normal and an abnormal blood pressure is not easy to define. Perhaps the best definition is the level of blood pressure above which treatment has been shown to be worthwhile (see p.21).

MEASURING BLOOD PRESSURE

Most people will have had their blood pressure taken at least once – perhaps by the doctor or nurse at the surgery, in hospital or, in the case of a pregnant woman, at the antenatal clinic. You may possibly have opted to have it done at a pharmacy or health food shop, or even have tried taking it yourself using one of the special kits that can be bought over the counter.

Although the ideal method would be to measure the blood pressure actually inside the arteries, this is clearly not feasible on a large scale because it would involve needles. However, an accurate reflection of the pressure under which blood is being pumped can be obtained using a less invasive approach.

The person performing the check wraps a rubber-lined cuff, which is part of the pressure-measuring device known as a sphygmomanometer, around your upper arm

Sphygmomanometer

The sphygmomanometer is the most common device
used to measure blood pressure. It consists of an
inflatable cuff attached to a tube containing mercury.
The blood pressure measurements are expressed in
millimetres of mercury.

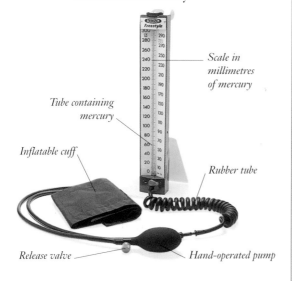

*Scale in
millimetres
of mercury*

*Tube containing
mercury*

Inflatable cuff

Rubber tube

Release valve

Hand-operated pump

and inflates it with a small hand pump to stop the blood
flow to your arm temporarily. The doctor or nurse then
puts a stethoscope over the artery just below the cuff
to listen to the sounds as the cuff is slowly deflated
and the blood flow returns to your arm.

When the cuff is blown up to a pressure between the
systolic and diastolic pressures, the blood in the artery
flows past for only part of each heartbeat; this intermittent flow causes the sounds. The pressure in the
cuff when the sounds first appear corresponds to the

13

systolic blood pressure. The disappearance of the sounds corre-sponds to the diastolic blood pressure, which is the pressure as the heart relaxes.

The sounds the doctor or nurse hears through the stethoscope are caused by turbulence of blood in the artery at the front of your elbow joint (the brachial pulse) and are referred to as Korotkoff sounds in honour of Russian army surgeon Nicholai Korotkoff, who first devised a system for listening to them in 1905.

A mercury gauge attached to the cuff allows the two pressures to be determined and recorded. The pressure applied within the arm cuff is measured in millimetres of mercury (mmHg), this being the height to which the mercury has to be pumped up in a glass tube.

Clearly, as this method of measuring blood pressure is indirect, it cannot be totally accurate and sometimes it may be very inaccurate, particularly in people who have very thick arms. If your arm circumference is more than 35 centimetres, the cuff will not cut off the circulation sufficiently when inflated, so the reading may be an overestimate of your true blood pressure. However, over the years it has become clear that this indirect way of measuring blood pressure is an accurate means of predicting an individual's chances of developing a heart attack or a stroke.

More recently, small, electronic, desktop systems that do not use mercury have been increasingly used for blood pressure measurement. However, many of these new blood pressure measurement machines are sadly rather inaccurate and very few are recommended by the British Hypertension Society. Although these machines do not use a column of mercury to measure the pressure, they still report the blood pressure in millimetres of mercury, simply so that the readings obtained are comparable to those from the mercury 'gold standard' system. It makes little difference which type of equipment is being used when you are having your blood pressure taken because the procedure involved is much the same.

Usually, you will be asked to sit down and the cuff is applied to your upper arm so that it is roughly at the same level as your heart. It is very important that you are as relaxed as possible and that your arm is supported by resting your elbow on a table – the effort of holding it up could otherwise produce a falsely high reading.

Everyone's blood pressure is immensely variable, and yours may go up if you are feeling anxious or stressed, so try to relax as much as possible while it is being measured. Your doctor or nurse will probably take the first reading as a rough guide and take a second measure-ment to get the actual reading. If your blood pressure is clearly settling to a lower level between the first and second reading, you may need to have a third or even a fourth reading at another visit to the clinic some days or weeks later to make sure the final figure is a truly representative value. This is particularly important if the finding on the first or second measurement is only slightly above normal. There is evidence to suggest that, in most people, the blood pressure 'bottoms-out' at the fourth visit, with little further fall after that, but there are exceptions to this rule.

TAKING BLOOD PRESSURE
A doctor uses a sphygmo-manometer to measure systolic and diastolic blood pressures.

With few exceptions, the blood pressure is the same in both arms, so it is best to use the nearest arm for convenience. It is sometimes a good idea to check both arms on one occasion to ensure that there is no systematic difference. If your upper arm is larger than average (more than 33 centimetres around), the person measuring your blood pressure will need to use a larger cuff, otherwise there may be a falsely high reading. About 15 per cent of people with high blood pressure have an arm circumference that is greater than 33 centimetres, so it is crucially important that the correct size of cuff is used.

Although it is not normal to be asked to stand up to have your blood pressure checked (because it is more difficult to provide support for your arm), there are occasions when it is done – for example, in some people with diabetes and in elderly people or anyone who experiences dizziness or other symptoms when standing up. The former is because the blood pressure of people with diabetes may fall briefly when they stand. Normally, there is no significant change in blood pressure on standing up but, in certain conditions, including diabetes, this can occur, and it is referred to as postural hypotension. It may or may not be associated with dizziness.

SYSTOLIC BLOOD PRESSURE

As we have seen, measuring blood pressure involves recording both the highest (systolic) and the lowest (diastolic) levels in your system, so the reading will record two figures. Conventionally, blood pressure is expressed as systolic pressure over diastolic pressure, for example 140/94 mmHg (millimetres of mercury).

The relative importance of systolic and diastolic blood pressure has been the subject of much research. In fact,

Blood Pressure Reading

Two readings are recorded when blood pressure is taken. Systolic blood pressure is the higher reading and diastolic blood pressure is the lower reading.

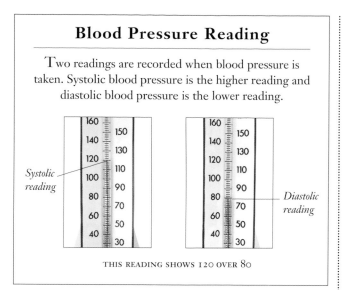

THIS READING SHOWS 120 OVER 80

contrary to what most people believe, once over the age of 40 systolic pressure is more important than diastolic when it comes to predicting who will get heart disease. The problem is that everyone's systolic blood pressure, and especially that of older people, varies considerably.

The importance of systolic blood pressure has recently been emphasised by the publication of two reliable studies that showed reducing the systolic pressure was worthwhile in people whose diastolic blood pressure was normal. This condition is known medically as isolated systolic hypertension (ISH). It mostly affects people over the age of 65 and, if it is not treated, they are at high risk of developing heart disease or stroke. In general, the lower your blood pressure, the better. When treating high blood pressure, the aim is to reduce all risk factors for heart disease, such as smoking, high cholesterol levels, etc., and to try to keep blood pressure under 140/90 mmHg.

'WHITE COAT' HYPERTENSION

'White coat' and 'office' hypertension are terms applied to those people whose blood pressure is raised only when they are seeing a doctor. In recent years, it has become possible to record blood pressure over 24–hour periods at home (using automatic electronic equipment), and this has shown that many people's blood pressure goes back down to the normal range within an hour or so of leaving the surgery or hospital. When this happens, the person is said to have 'white coat' hypertension. The technique used for detecting 'white coat' hypertension is called ambulatory blood pressure monitoring (ABPM).

The exact significance of 'white coat' hypertension remains uncertain, but the current evidence suggests that people with this condition cannot be considered to be entirely healthy. There is evidence that they are more likely to have enlargement of their heart than people with normal blood pressure. Furthermore, they may well develop sustained (or fixed) hypertension within five years, and they will then need treatment to lower their blood pressure.

This means that, although people with 'white coat' hypertension do not need treatment immediately, they do need to have regular blood pressure checks every six or 12 months.

It is also true that many people who do have genuine hypertension that requires treatment also have a large 'white coat effect'. Thus, when they are away from the surgery or hospital, their pressures are much lower and the doctor needs to take this into account when deciding how much medication they need to take to control their blood pressure.

HOME MEASUREMENTS

If it is necessary for you to have your blood pressure measured away from the hospital or clinic, there are several ways that this can be done:

- You may be provided with a conventional mercury blood pressure machine and a stethoscope and shown how to use them, but this is not entirely satisfactory and it can be rather awkward.
- A relative can be shown how to measure your blood pressure and this may provide useful information.
- You may be advised to buy one of the newer and relatively inexpensive electronic automatic blood pressure machines, although many of these are as yet not very accurate. The best buys are easy to use, easy to read, cheap and portable. (To date, only the Omron M4 apparatus has passed the British Hypertension Society's tests for accuracy.) All you have to do is place the cuff around your arm then press a button. You can take as many readings as necessary, and this can provide useful information for your doctor, so long as the machine is accurate. If you do buy one of these simple desktop blood pressure machines, you will probably be advised to take it into the hospital, clinic or health centre so that the doctor or the nurse can quickly check the accuracy of the equipment against the mercury blood pressure 'gold standard'.

SELF-MEASUREMENT
You can use a conventional blood pressure machine to measure your blood pressure at home, but it can be difficult to get an accurate reading.

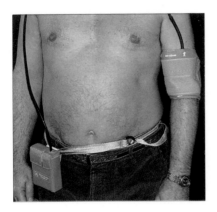

A 24–HOUR RECORD
An ambulatory monitor can be worn both day and night to repeatedly record a person's blood pressure.

● In some cases, your doctor may set up a home measuring system with an automatic 24–hour ambulatory blood pressure monitor (ABPM). Several reliable and accurate systems are now available that can be programmed to measure the blood pressure every half hour or so over 24 hours. Perhaps surprisingly, using these machines at night does not often cause any sleep disturbance. The value of 24–hour ambulatory blood pressure monitoring still remains a little controversial, but it is an accurate method of obtaining information that will help the doctor to decide whether you have any degree of 'white coat' hypertension.

KEY POINTS

● High blood pressure is caused by a narrowing of the microscopic arterioles in all tissues.

● Systolic pressure is the pressure in the larger vessels when the heart contracts.

● Diastolic pressure is the pressure when the heart relaxes between beats.

● It is important that you are totally relaxed when your blood pressure is being measured.

● Systolic blood pressure is now known to be as important as, or even more important than, diastolic pressure.

● Automatic measuring systems can be employed to measure blood pressure away from the clinic or health centre.

What is hypertension?

If your blood pressure reading is consistently over 160/90 mmHg, you will be told that you have hypertension, but, generally speaking, the lower your blood pressure, the better. If your pressure is between 140/90 and 160/90 mmHg, then you may be diagnosed as having 'borderline' hypertension.

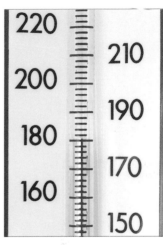

Blood pressure readings are a remarkably accurate predictor of life expectancy: the higher the pressure the greater the risk. Even people whose blood pressures are average for the population have a slightly greater risk of heart disease than people with lower than average levels. For this reason, it has been extremely difficult to find a simple working definition of hypertension. Perhaps the most sensible view is to define it as 'that level of blood pressure where treatment with antihypertensive drugs does more good than harm', because there is no such thing as drug treatment that does not have some potential side-effects.

If your blood pressure is found to be more than 160/90 mmHg, and if you have several different risk

A HIGH READING
If the blood pressure monitor reveals a reading of over 160/90 mmHg, you are considered to be suffering from hypertension.

factors for heart disease, such as high cholesterol, being a smoker and a family tendency to heart disease, then treating your high blood pressure is likely to be very worthwhile. (This is explained in detail in the section beginning on p.46.)

On the other hand, for some young people with only very marginally raised blood pressure, and no other risk factors for heart disease, the value of blood pressure-lowering drugs is very small and drug treatment may therefore be held back. It is, however, crucial that such people are re-checked at intervals of roughly about six months.

Hypertension has been called the 'silent killer' because it usually causes no symptoms until a late stage of the disease. Contrary to what many people believe, it is not possible to feel your own blood pressure. The only way to find out whether your blood pressure is raised is to have it measured with a blood pressure machine (see p.12).

As hypertension causes no symptoms until complications begin to show themselves, about half of all individuals who have it remain unaware that they have a problem.

══ WHY HYPERTENSION MATTERS ══

Blood vessels are like rubber tubes that carry blood constantly to wherever it is needed. Arteries, which carry blood out of the heart, have to withstand the great pressures with which the blood is pumped out. If the blood pressure is higher than usual over many years, as in untreated hypertension, the vessels become damaged. The lining of the arteries can become roughened and thickened, and this eventually causes them to narrow and become less flexible, or elastic, than previously. This is

What Happens to Damaged Blood Vessels?

The process of thrombosis (blood clot formation) may be triggered by damage to the lining of a blood vessel as a result of hypertension. The resulting clot may then obstruct the flow of blood through the vessel.

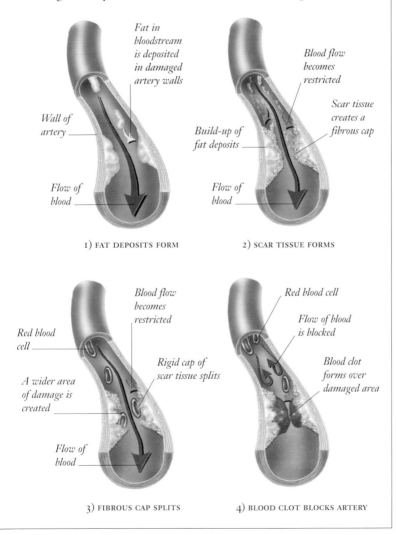

Fat in bloodstream is deposited in damaged artery walls

Wall of artery

Flow of blood

1) FAT DEPOSITS FORM

Blood flow becomes restricted

Scar tissue creates a fibrous cap

Build-up of fat deposits

Flow of blood

2) SCAR TISSUE FORMS

Blood flow becomes restricted

Red blood cell

A wider area of damage is created

Rigid cap of scar tissue splits

Flow of blood

3) FIBROUS CAP SPLITS

Red blood cell

Flow of blood is blocked

Blood clot forms over damaged area

4) BLOOD CLOT BLOCKS ARTERY

23

Risk Factors for Coronary Heart Disease

Several factors have been found to influence an individual's risk of developing coronary heart disease. The greater the number of risk factors that apply to you, the greater your chance of developing CHD.

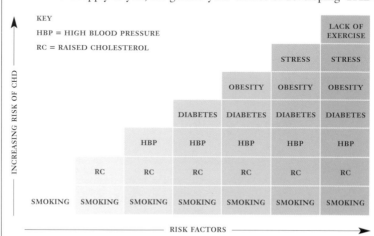

KEY

HBP = HIGH BLOOD PRESSURE

RC = RAISED CHOLESTEROL

INCREASING RISK OF CHD

						LACK OF EXERCISE
					STRESS	STRESS
				OBESITY	OBESITY	OBESITY
			DIABETES	DIABETES	DIABETES	DIABETES
		HBP	HBP	HBP	HBP	HBP
	RC	RC	RC	RC	RC	RC
SMOKING	SMOKING	SMOKING	SMOKING	SMOKING	SMOKING	SMOKING

RISK FACTORS

known as arteriosclerosis. If an artery becomes too narrow, blood cannot get through properly, and the part of the body that relies on that artery for its blood supply is starved of blood and the all-important oxygen that it carries. As the artery narrows there is an increased tendency to develop blood clots (thrombosis), which may cause total blockage of the artery so that the part of the body that it serves dies. If the heart or the brain is affected, the dead area is called an infarct.

OTHER RISK FACTORS

High blood pressure over many years can cause all these problems, and the whole point of measuring blood pressure regularly, and treating it effectively if it is high, is to prevent these complications. However, you are more likely to develop these complications if you smoke and if you have untreated high blood cholesterol levels. The reason is that cigarette smoking damages blood vessels in much the same way as high blood pressure, making the artery itself narrower and its lining thick and rough. High cholesterol can cause fatty deposits, called atheroma, in the lining of the artery to develop more rapidly than normal, which also helps to narrow the arteries. It is not possible for your level of serum cholesterol to be too low, and treatment to lower cholesterol saves lives.

Another common risk factor that can also contribute to narrowing of the arteries, known as cardiovascular disease, is diabetes (diabetes mellitus), which affects four to five per cent of the white population and 10–15 per cent of the south Asian and Afro-Caribbean population in the UK. High glucose levels in the blood damage arteries in a similar way to high blood pressure.

But it would not do to paint too gloomy a picture. The whole point of having your blood pressure checked is that, if you are found to have hypertension, it is possible to treat it effectively and so bring your risk of heart disease and strokes back down to normal. It does not matter particularly how severe the hypertension was in the first place. What is really important is how well your blood pressure is controlled over the ensuing years.

It is better to have had severe hypertension that has been well treated than to have slightly raised blood pressure that remains untreated or neglected.

Long-term Effects of High Blood Pressure

Although there are many serious long-term effects of high blood pressure, it must be stressed that all of these complications can be prevented with effective antihypertensive treatment.

- The heart is a muscle that needs its own blood supply, which is brought to it by the coronary arteries. If these arteries narrow, blood does not get to the heart muscle efficiently. So when the heart needs to work a bit harder than usual, e.g. when you are walking up a hill, the heart muscle cannot get the blood supply and oxygen that it needs. This causes pain in the chest, known as myocardial ischaemia or angina.

- If a coronary artery narrows and then a blood clot forms, the part of the heart muscle that relies on that coronary artery dies. This is known as a coronary thrombosis, a myocardial infarction or a heart attack.

- Over the years, as arteries narrow and become less elastic as a result of hypertension, it gets harder and harder for the heart to pump blood out efficiently to the rest of the body. The increased workload eventually damages the heart and impairs its performance. Fluid collects in the lungs, causing shortness of breath. This is known as congestive cardiac failure, or heart failure.

- Narrowing of an artery that carries blood and oxygen to the brain can lead to temporary loss of function in the part of the brain served by that artery; this is known as a transient ischaemic attack (TIA). Permanent closing off of the artery with a blood clot results in the death of the part of the brain reliant on that artery, which results in a stroke.

- Smaller blood vessels in the legs can be damaged, resulting in less blood getting to the feet, and pain in the calf muscles on walking.

- When blood vessels supplying the kidneys are affected, the result may be gradual kidney damage. This is why a blood test to check kidney function is a vital part of regular check-ups for anyone with hypertension.

- The small blood vessels in the eyes can also be affected, although this may not become apparent until damage is extensive. Rarely, in severe hypertension, there may be damage to the retina with haemorrhages. This condition is called malignant hypertension, although with treatment the outlook is very good.

KEY POINTS

- High blood pressure is one of the three main risk factors for heart attack and stroke.

- The other risk factors are smoking and raised blood cholesterol levels.

- Lowering blood pressure (and lowering blood cholesterol) saves lives.

What causes hypertension?

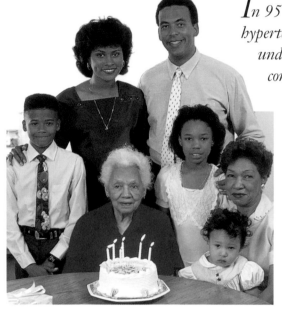

IN THE FAMILY
Genetic factors may increase your chance of having high blood pressure. People of Afro-Caribbean origin are particularly susceptible to hypertension.

In 95 per cent of cases of hypertension there is no specific underlying cause, and this condition is known as primary, or essential, hypertension. The remaining five per cent of people have a problem with their kidneys or with the small glands known as the adrenals. Doctors refer to this as secondary hypertension.

A number of factors may contribute to hypertension. Heredity plays a part, which means that hypertension can run in families. Blood pressure tends to increase with age, but this is partly because of changes in lifestyle; many people put on weight and get less active as they get older, and both these factors may contribute to the development of hypertension. More importantly, the rise in blood pressure with age is greater in people who eat a lot of salty foods.

Racial background plays a part, with people of Afro-Caribbean origin living in Western societies having a higher prevalence of hypertension than white people. This is probably because Afro-Caribbean people handle salt in the body differently. However, migration studies show that, although racial origins do play a part, it is the diet and other lifestyle factors that are more significant. Someone who lives in a more affluent Western country is more prone to hypertension than someone who lives in a poorer country.

Blood pressure always varies throughout the day and is usually higher during exercise as the heart needs to pump blood around the body faster, although people who exercise regularly will tend to have lower blood pressures than non-active people when at rest. Your blood pressure is lower when you are sleeping or resting. But you will not be diagnosed as having hypertension on the basis of a one-off reading. You will need to have at least two high (i.e. over 160/90 mmHg) readings on three separate occasions, over at least two months. Ideally, your blood pressure should be checked sitting down, as rested and relaxed as possible. If your blood pressure is dangerously high or in special circumstances – for example, if you are pregnant – more urgent measures may be needed.

REGULATING BLOOD PRESSURE

There are two systems in the body that are involved in helping us to maintain normal blood pressure in all circumstances if possible. One is the sympathetic nervous system, which releases chemicals such as adrenaline and noradrenaline; these can both open blood vessels (vasodilate) and close them (vasoconstrict)

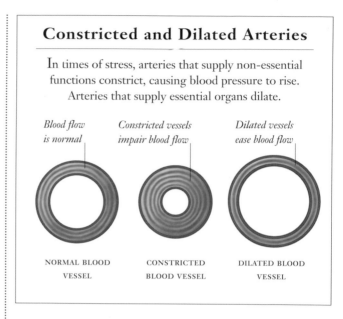

Constricted and Dilated Arteries

In times of stress, arteries that supply non-essential functions constrict, causing blood pressure to rise. Arteries that supply essential organs dilate.

Blood flow is normal

Constricted vessels impair blood flow

Dilated vessels ease blood flow

NORMAL BLOOD VESSEL

CONSTRICTED BLOOD VESSEL

DILATED BLOOD VESSEL

as required, depending on which parts of our body need to be ready for action. This system comes into operation to enable us to respond in a crisis by concentrating our physical resources where they are needed in order to help us to survive a perceived threat. This means shutting down the body's non-essential functions – such as digestion – for the duration of the crisis to prepare us for 'fight or flight'. For early humans, this was essential when life was full of physical danger, but for most people today the system is most likely to be triggered by emotional or psychological stress rather than by actual life-threatening situations. As a result of its narrowing effect on small blood vessels, this process can play a part in causing hypertension. Drugs that act on this system, for example beta-blockers such as atenolol, can therefore be used to control it.

The other important system is a hormone produced by the kidneys, known as renin, which activates an enzyme called angiotensin II. Angiotensin II makes blood vessels constrict. Drugs that block angiotensin, called angiotensin-converting enzyme (ACE) inhibitors, such as enalapril, can help to lower hypertension. Angio-tensin also stimulates the release of a hormone called aldosterone from the adrenal glands. This hormone causes salt and water retention by the kidneys and may further elevate the blood pressure.

The microscopic blood vessels, called arterioles, have smooth muscle cells in their walls that contract when calcium concentrations rise. People with hypertension have higher calcium levels in their smooth muscle cells than those with normal blood pressure, although it is still not known why. In people with hypertension, it is

How ACE Inhibitor Drugs Work

ACE inhibitors work by blocking the action of an enzyme in the blood that is responsible for converting angiotensin I into angiotensin II, which causes the blood vessels to constrict. ACE inhibitors therefore keep the blood vessels dilated.

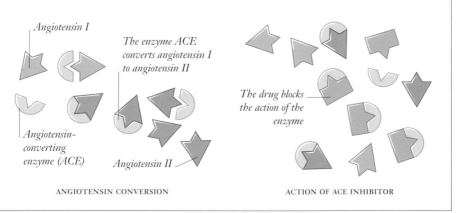

Angiotensin I

The enzyme ACE converts angiotensin I to angiotensin II

The drug blocks the action of the enzyme

Angiotensin-converting enzyme (ACE)

Angiotensin II

ANGIOTENSIN CONVERSION

ACTION OF ACE INHIBITOR

thought that these rises in the calcium concentration cause the arterioles to contract, which makes it harder for the heart to pump blood through them. Long-term contraction of the arterioles is also thought to damage their walls, leading to further rises in blood pressure as the smooth flow of blood is disturbed. Drugs that block the calcium channels (calcium antagonists, such as nifedipine) allow the arterioles to open up again, which lowers blood pressure.

Although all the hormones mentioned here (renin, angiotensin, aldosterone, adrenaline and noradrenaline) play a role in regulating blood pressure in all people, it seems that people with high blood pressure are more susceptible to them. People with hypertension do not have more of these hormones in their bloodstream, but blocking their effects with drugs lowers blood pressure only if it was raised in the first place.

The final common pathway of all of these mechanisms is narrowing of the arterioles, causing increased resistance to blood flow. The heart continues to pump normally, so the pressure within the whole arterial system rises.

LIFESTYLE FACTORS

As far as you as an individual are concerned, your blood pressure level depends on the interplay of genetic or inherited factors and the influences of your lifestyle. Hypertension clearly runs in families, and this holds true even after allowances have been made for the fact that families tend to share the same lifestyle and diet. Excellent research conducted among twins who were brought up separately or together, and also among adopted children compared with non-adopted children, has been able to identify how much of the similarity in blood pressure within families is the result of inher itance compared with the proportion resulting from similarities in lifestyle. Roughly speaking, about half of all the variation in blood pressure between people is the result of genetic factors and half is the result of dietary factors dating back to early childhood.

SALT INTAKE

Salt intake has a direct effect on blood pressure. It has been shown that the rise in blood pressure as we get older, which occurs in all urban societies, is the result in large measure of the amount of salt we eat. Reducing salt intake helps to reduce blood pressure. A high salt intake over many years probably raises blood pressure by raising the sodium content of the smooth muscle cells of the walls of the arterioles. This high sodium content appears to facilitate the entry of calcium into the cells; this in turn causes them to contract and narrow the internal diameter of the arteriole.

SALT AND HYPERTENSION
Salt consumption is certainly a factor in high blood pressure. The recommended daily intake of salt is less than 5 grams – about a teaspoonful – but in the UK the average intake in men is twice this.

There is some evidence that people with an inherited tendency to develop hypertension have a reduced capacity to remove salt from their bodies. There is, however, little evidence that such people consume more salt than anyone else, although they may tend to retain what they do eat.

The relationship between salt and hypertension has, over the years, been controversial, mainly because the original research was not carried out carefully enough. However, during the mid-1980s a very reliable international comparative study convincingly showed that there is a close relationship between salt intake and blood pressure when comparing people in different countries.

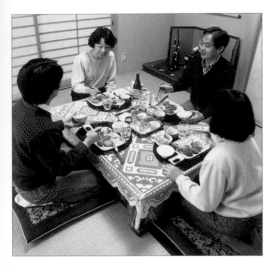

CULTURAL DIFFERENCES
The Japanese diet tends to be high in salt – contained in such things as fish and soy sauce – and this helps to explain the high incidence of hypertension in Japan.

For instance, the Japanese, Polish and Portuguese have a high salt intake and a high frequency of raised blood pressure and strokes. Furthermore, it was found that those populations that have a large amount of salt in their diet are also those populations in which blood pressure rises with advancing age. By contrast, populations in which salt intake is low show only a small rise in blood pressure with advancing age and therefore hypertension is relatively less common. As we will discuss later in this book, there is now good evidence that reducing the amount of salt in the diet does lower blood pressure. It is certainly true, however, that there are variations in the way individuals' bodies handle salt and some people are more sensitive to it than others. This is probably true of people with a strong family history of hypertension, and it is also evident that older people are more salt-sensitive, as are people who are of Afro-Caribbean origin.

The relationship between salt intake and the subsequent development of hypertension has recently been confirmed by an extremely reliable study that began by looking at babies who were weaned either on to a low-salt diet or a normal-salt diet. After six months, blood pressure was significantly better (lower) in the low-salt babies. A proportion of these babies has now been followed up for 15 years, and their blood pressures were found to be still significantly lower.

If children could be persuaded to consume less salt then we might prevent the development of hypertension in the first place, which means we should be seriously concerned about the amount of salt in crisps and other snacks that children nowadays consume in large quantities.

WEIGHT

Overweight people tend to have higher blood pressure than thin people. This is partly because obese people's bodies have to work harder to burn up the excess calories they consume, partly because they tend to eat more salt than normal and possibly because fat people have a tendency to be resistant to the hormone insulin, which deals with blood sugars, and this may be involved in causing high blood pressure, although it is not yet fully understood.

Although overweight people do appear to have higher blood pressure than people of normal weight, this may in part be related to a tendency for doctors and nurses using conventional blood pressure machines to over-estimate their blood pressure. The greater the circum-ference of the upper arm where the blood pressure cuff is applied, the greater the over-estimation of blood pressure. This can partly be overcome if they make sure they use a larger arm cuff when appropriate. However, even when allowances have been made for this tendency to overestimate blood pressure, there is still a convincing relationship between body weight and blood pressure.

It is not possible to say whether you are overweight just on the basis of how much you actually weigh (because tall people usually weigh more than short people), so instead doctors usually work out what is called the body mass index (BMI). This is calculated by taking your weight in kilograms and dividing it by the square of your

Are You a Healthy Weight?

To find out whether you are a healthy weight for your height, first find your current weight on the left side of the chart below. Then run your finger across to your height and see which of the three sections you fall into.

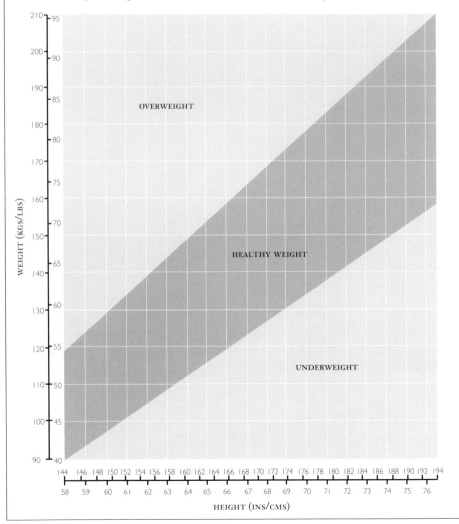

height in metres. This can be shown by the mathematical equation BMI = [Weight (kg)]/[Height (m)]^2.

A person who has a body mass index of 30 or more is considered obese, whereas if BMI is between 25 and 30 he or she would be considered to be slightly overweight.

Population surveys have shown that the variation in blood pressure between people in relation to their weight is about one millimetre of mercury (mmHg) per kilogram (or two pounds) in weight. When you put on weight, the amount you gain is a good guide to the amount by which your blood pressure will rise. If you lose weight, your blood pressure will fall by an amount that can be predicted using the same formula.

The relationship between body weight and blood pressure is more complex than was originally thought, and it may also be related to important effects of certain hormones, as well as to the body's capacity to handle salt. From a practical point of view, however, losing weight is a very effective way of reducing your blood pressure.

ALCOHOL

Alcohol has an effect on blood pressure and, on the whole, the more alcohol you drink the higher your blood pressure, although it is not understood why. Interestingly, teetotallers tend to have slightly higher blood pressures than moderate drinkers – so two glasses of wine or a pint of beer a day may be better for you than none at all by helping to protect you against heart disease.

Heavy drinkers or alcoholics are very likely to have raised blood pressure and also have a strong tendency to develop strokes. When such people stop drinking their blood pressure comes down.

Recognising a Unit of Alcohol

Drinks contain different amounts of alcohol. Weekly intake should not exceed 21 units for men and 14 units for women. A unit of alcohol is equivalent to approximately 8–10 grams of pure alcohol.

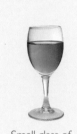

Small glass of sherry = 1 unit

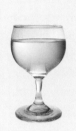

Small glass of wine = 1 unit

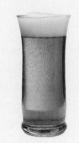

½ pint of beer or cider, or ¼ pint of strong lager = 1 unit

Single measure of aperitif or spirit = 1 unit

Although the relationship between alcohol and blood pressure is now well recognised, no one has yet discovered a convincing mechanism to explain how this happens. However, doctors recommend that men should drink no more than 21 units of alcohol per week (equivalent to 10½ pints of beer or 21 small glasses of wine) and women should drink no more than 14 units per week (equivalent to seven pints of beer or 14 small glasses of wine). These should be spread over the week, not drunk all at once.

STRESS
Stress can raise your blood pressure in the short term, but it probably does not account for long-term rises in blood pressure. Relaxation techniques may help to improve your quality of life, but probably will not be enough to control true hypertension.

The relationship between stress and blood pressure is confusing, and much of the earlier research in this field was not satisfactory by modern standards. There is no doubt that acutely stressful stimuli can cause a dramatic rise in blood pressure. For example, if you are given some extremely bad or distressing news, your blood pressure may be raised soon afterwards. Similarly, in experimental situations the stress of conducting mental arithmetic in a noisy environment, or even sorting out different-sized objects, causes a sudden sharp rise in blood pressure.

If going to see a doctor, whether it is your GP or a doctor in a hospital clinic, makes you feel anxious and nervous, your blood pressure is likely to go up. For this reason, you should be asked to come back and have it measured again on several occasions if it is slightly raised on your first visit. The idea is that, once you have become more familiar with the environment and the procedure, you will be better able to relax and the reading will then be a more accurate reflection of your blood pressure when you are not under any stress.

Although the effects of this kind of short-term stress on blood pressure are well recognised, there is little evidence that chronic (that is, long-term) stress causes chronic hypertension. Reliable studies have shown no relationship between levels of stress, as assessed by detailed and accurate questioning, and blood pressure. People with very stressful jobs do not have more hypertension or heart disease than people with less stressful jobs. However, the research in this field has been seriously hampered by the lack of reliable measures of stress, so the subject remains somewhat controversial.

There is some evidence that people who have less control over their day-to-day life at work have higher

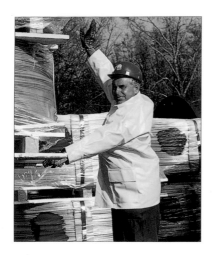

blood pressures than people who can influence their working lives more effectively. Thus manual workers tend to have higher blood pressures than executives or managers. The differences between these groups, however, are also related to differences in lifestyle and diet, and it is difficult to be sure how much of these differences is the result of stress alone.

POTASSIUM AND CALCIUM

Eating lots of foods that contain potassium – such as fruit and vegetables – is good for keeping blood pressure low. However, people with high-potassium diets often have a fairly low salt intake, so it is hard to know whether it is the low salt or the high potassium that is helping. That said, potassium does seem to be beneficial in its own right. There is quite good evidence that people who have a low-potassium diet have higher blood pressure, whereas those who eat a lot of fruit and vegetables have lower blood pressure and a lower incidence of stroke. This makes sense because we know that cells respond to high potassium by getting rid of sodium (in salt).

This effect of potassium intake is small compared with that of salt. However, it is true to say that variations in salt intake between people are also associated with parallel variations in potassium intake. As already stated, people who eat a lot of potassium-rich foods generally eat relatively little salt, whereas salt fans tend to eat less fruit and vegetables.

There has been some research to suggest that a diet high in calcium may be protective against hypertension.

However, these results are highly controversial and at the present state of knowledge no recommendations can be made on changing the diet accordingly.

It is clear that there are many nutritional factors that influence blood pressure and these are the subject of a major research project, which was started in 1997. It is likely therefore that we will have more information some time after the year 2000.

EXERCISE

Although your blood pressure rises sharply while you are actually exercising, if you exercise regularly you will tend to be healthier and have lower blood pressure than people who do not take any exercise. This is partly because people who exercise are more likely to eat healthily, not smoke and not drink excessive alcohol, although exercise also seems to have a direct effect on lowering blood pressure. You should aim to take regular, moderate amounts of exercise rather than going in for very vigorous bouts every now and again.

SYMPTOMS

The vast majority of people with hypertension have no symptoms. Some people believe that they can feel their blood pressure but, in fact, it is more likely that they are feeling emotional stress, for example of attending hospital or some recent stressful event in their home life. This short-term stress may or may not raise blood pressure.

The fact that hypertension causes no symptoms means that it is often not diagnosed for many years, by which time the person has subtle evidence of damage to his or her heart, brain or kidneys. At a later stage, they may go to their doctor because they have started to feel unwell.

They may, for example, have had a small stroke or have angina (chest pain on exertion), or they may even have had a heart attack. Someone who has developed heart failure may feel breathless when lying down, whereas kidney failure can be responsible for general tiredness and exhaustion as well as breathlessness.

These are serious problems, which is why you should never wait until you feel ill before having your blood pressure checked. The current opinion is that everyone over the age of 30 should have a routine blood pressure check by their GP. The likelihood is that your reading will be normal or require no action and, if so, you probably only need to be re-checked every three or four years, but some people with borderline pressures may need to be checked more often.

INCIDENCE OF HYPERTENSION

The answer to the question of how common hypertension is clearly depends on the criteria used for diagnosis. Hypertension is more common with advancing age, particularly in populations who have a high salt intake, so age must be taken into account when we consider the prevalence of hypertension. Premenopausal women tend to have lower blood pressures than men of the same age, although the difference between the sexes becomes less apparent over the age of 50 years.

This is because, before the menopause, women are relatively protected from heart disease by the female hormone oestrogen. Oestrogen levels fall after the menopause and women start to catch up with men in terms of developing heart disease.

Any dividing line between so-called high blood pressure and normal blood pressure must be purely arbitrary.

Even if your blood pressure is around the average for the population as a whole, you are at higher risk than someone whose blood pressure is persistently below this level. Thus a blood pressure of 140/80 mmHg carries a slightly worse prognosis than a blood pressure of 130/70 mmHg. As explained on p.21, the most useful definition of hypertension is therefore that level of blood pressure where treatment is necessary to prevent the individual developing heart disease, strokes and other complications of hypertension.

At the present state of knowledge, on the basis of reliable trials of the drug treatment of hypertension

Who Gets Hypertension?

This chart shows hypertension in people 20 years of age and over according to sex. The increasing incidence of hypertension as we grow older is clearly shown in these graphs.

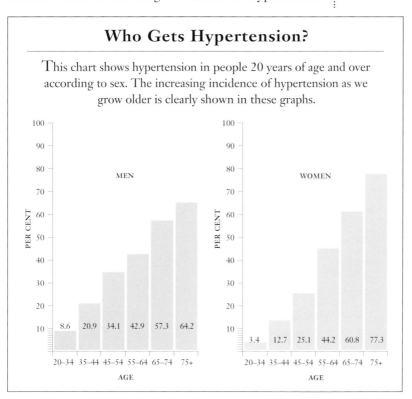

compared with placebo (dummy) tablets, we know that treatment is necessary if blood pressure is consistently 160/90 mmHg or more at all ages.

Around 25 per cent of people have a diastolic blood pressure of 90 mmHg or more, although it is worth stressing that many of them will have a lower reading on re-checking so no treatment may be necessary. Should the level not fall when your blood pressure is measured again, you may need drug treatment. If your diastolic pressure is below 90 mmHg, but your systolic pressure is over 160 mmHg, you will be diagnosed as having isolated systolic hypertension (ISH). This condition is very rare in people under the age of 60 but affects 20–30 per cent of those over the age of 80. Recent research has shown that treatment to lower the systolic pressure is very effective at preventing heart attacks and strokes.

If we take into consideration all types of hypertension affecting people over the age of 60, about 35–40 per cent of men and women in the UK need further assessment on the basis of either a raised diastolic or a raised systolic pressure. However, this percentage is lower among people whose consumption of salt is below the national average.

Surveys suggest that between seven and 10 million people in the UK have raised blood pressure levels. Socioeconomic factors seem to play a part – people who live in poorer areas of the UK are more likely to have hypertension than those who live in more affluent areas. Certainly, heart disease and strokes are more prevalent in the north and north-west of England, and in Scotland, than in the south-east of England, although this also reflects smoking habits.

It must be stressed that many of these pressures are only slightly raised and will be lower on re-checking.

Estimates of the number of people with raised blood pressure who require drug treatment vary between 10 and 15 per cent of the adult population. This represents a very small proportion of people aged 20–30 years but about half of those over the age of 70. Hypertension is therefore the most common chronic, that is non-infective, medical condition in the western world. About 50 million people in the USA have blood pressure levels that require treatment, and a similar figure is seen in studies from the European Union. The prevalence of hypertension in the UK is higher than in France, Italy, Spain and Greece, and similar to that seen in Sweden and Denmark. In both the UK and the USA, however, hypertension is much more common in people of African origin. The reasons for this are not entirely clear, but it is possible that these people tend to handle the salt in their diet in a different way, so that their bodies retain more of it, and this puts their blood pressure up. For more on this, see p.34.

KEY POINTS

- Hypertension runs in families.
- Hypertension is related to a high salt intake, being overweight and drinking too much alcohol.
- Rarely, high blood pressure is the result of underlying kidney disease or excess of certain hormones.

How hypertension is investigated

If you are found to have hypertension, your doctor will give you a detailed physical examination and arrange for you to have a number of tests. These may include blood and urine tests and an electro-cardiogram (ECG). More severe cases of hypertension may be referred to a specialist hospital clinic for further tests.

There are three principal reasons why you may need to have tests and investigations if you are found to have raised blood pressure levels:

VISITING THE DOCTOR
Your doctor will give you a full examination, including feeling your chest and tummy, if you are found to have hypertension.

- To check your cholesterol levels. If you have a high blood cholesterol level as well as hypertension, your risk of developing heart disease and strokes (cardiovascular risk) is correspondingly greater, and you will need treatment to bring both blood pressure and cholesterol levels back down to normal.

- To check for serious underlying disease. Occasionally, hypertension may be caused by certain kidney diseases and some extremely rare diseases of the adrenal glands, which are situated above each kidney.

• To check for heart and kidney damage. This may occur after prolonged untreated hypertension, so blood tests are taken to measure kidney function, and an electrocardiogram (ECG) is carried out to see if the heart is affected.

ROUTINE TESTS

All people with raised blood pressure need a simple urine test; a small blood specimen is also taken, and usually an ECG is done. First, however, you will be weighed and, if necessary, given advice on how to lose weight, which is likely to help reduce your blood pressure. Next, your doctor will examine your heart, chest, tummy and the pulses in your legs. This may give some indication as to whether hypertension has affected your heart or kidneys.

The type of heart damage called heart failure results in fluid retention that causes fluid on the lungs, which can be heard through a stethoscope. It can also cause an enlarged left side of the heart, which the doctor can detect.

Kidney damage can be diagnosed only by urine and blood tests.

If your hypertension is very severe, the doctor will probably use an instrument called an ophthalmoscope to look at the back of each eye (the retina) where it is possible to assess the tiny blood vessels. In mild hypertension, these blood vessels show only very minor changes, but in very severe hypertension there may be haemorrhages on the retina and areas of damage referred to as 'cottonwool spots'.

After the clinical examination, you will probably be asked to produce a small specimen of urine for testing.

Small arterioles

Veins

EFFECTS ON THE EYE
This view of the retina of a patient with hypertension shows that the small arterioles (pale red) are dilated and are restricting blood flow in the veins where they cross them.

If sugar is found in the urine this raises the possibility that you may have diabetes; if protein is found in the urine it could mean that you have some form of kidney condition. Blood tests are taken to measure your cholesterol level and to test the function of your kidneys. If the kidneys are not working properly, levels of urea and creatinine in the blood start to rise. In addition, levels of sodium and potassium in the blood are measured. These are abnormal in people whose hypertension is due to retained sodium because of the presence of a small benign tumour of the adrenal gland; this condition is called Conn's syndrome.

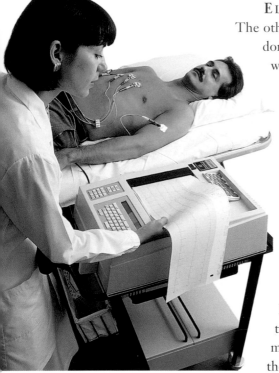

Having an ECG
To make an ECG recording, electrodes (conducting plates) are attached to the skin to make an electrical circuit with the ECG machine. The pattern of electrical impulses in the heart is recorded on a moving strip of paper.

ELECTROCARDIOGRAM
The other routine investigation that is usually done is an electrocardiogram, or ECG, which gives a recording of the electrical activity of the heart.

An electrocardiogram has a dual purpose. First, it can provide an indirect index of the size of the heart. When the blood pressure is very high, the heart enlarges in order to cope with increased load and this leads to increased voltages on the ECG. This is called left ventricular hypertrophy (or LVH) and is very important. When someone is found to have left ventricular hypertrophy, their need for treatment to lower their blood pressure becomes more urgent because it indicates that the heart muscle is under significant strain trying to cope with the effort of pumping blood round the body at increased pressure.

The second reason for doing an ECG is because it may show changes suggestive of narrowing or blockage of the coronary arteries, which supply the heart muscle. This process is called 'ischaemia' and is seen in some people who experience angina (chest pain) on exertion. Even though you may never have had symptoms of angina and have no reason to think you have ever suffered a heart attack, you may nevertheless show signs of ischaemic changes, and these are important to note.

FURTHER TESTS

Virtually everyone with hypertension will need the routine investigations above. You will require the more detailed investigations, which are usually done in hospital outpatient clinics, only if your hypertension is severe or if your doctor suspects that you have some underlying condition that is responsible for your blood pressure problems.

Two or three per cent of people with hypertension are found to have underlying medical conditions that cause their blood pressure to rise. These are diseases of the kidney and of the adrenal gland. In either case, you will probably be referred to a specialist clinic in your local hospital.

A further three or four per cent of people have very severe hypertension that needs more detailed investigation and care by a specialist in high blood pressure.

The vast majority of people with hypertension do not and should not attend hospital for their hypertension and can be cared for by their GP. There will be marked variations in the proportion of patients referred to hospital clinics, depending on the availability of local services and specialist blood pressure doctors. Whether you have to attend a hospital clinic will depend on your individual GP's policy in such cases. Some may refer a large number of their patients to be seen only once or twice for a full assessment in hospital and then look after them themselves, whereas others refer only very difficult cases to a hospital specialist.

VISITING A HOSPITAL CLINIC

Only a small minority of people with hypertension will need to attend hospital-based specialist clinics. As explained on p.49, these will usually be people whose hypertension is associated with complications such as heart disease or kidney disease, those whose blood pressure is proving difficult to control or those whose GP suspects that they may have some underlying condition that is causing their hypertension.

Suspicion of there being some underlying cause for the hypertension would be based on the presence of protein in the urine or abnormal blood test results, showing evidence of impairment of kidney function. In addition, if levels of potassium in the blood are found to be low, this raises the possibility that there may be an underlying disorder of the adrenal glands.

You will also be referred to a hospital clinic if your blood pressure varies greatly from minute to minute or hour to hour or even day to day. There is an extremely rare condition called phaeochromocytoma that is caused by the intermittent secretion of large quantities of adrenaline and noradrenaline by a tumour of the adrenal gland. When you do go to a clinic, you may have to undergo a repetition of some of the blood tests already done by your GP merely to confirm abnormalities. If there is a suspicion that you may have Conn's syndrome, in which hypertension is the result of an excess of a hormone called aldosterone, the hospital doctor may opt to measure this in your blood.

To exclude any form of kidney disease, it is usual to do an ultrasound scan to investigate the size and shape of the kidneys. This test is increasingly becoming a routine investigation for severely hypertensive people because it is safe and causes no discomfort. You may also be asked to provide a 24-hour collection of urine so that your body's 24-hour output of adrenaline and nora-drenaline can be measured. Raised levels could indicate that you have a phaeochromocytoma.

The clinic doctor may also measure your heart size by means of an echocardiogram, which is a type of ultrasound heart scan. Very often, people are referred to a hospital clinic because their blood pressure is proving a little resistant to treatment, and the hospital doctor may therefore opt to alter drug combinations and formulations in order to obtain better blood pressure control.

Once your blood pressure is under control and things are sorted out, you will normally be discharged from the care of the clinic back to your GP and have to go back to the hospital only if problems arise.

KEY POINTS

- All people diagnosed as hypertensive should have a spot urine check, a blood test and an ECG.
- Only a minority of patients need referral to specialist clinics for hypertension for further investigation.

Treatment without drugs

Treating hypertension without the use of drugs is sometimes called 'non-pharmacological' blood pressure reduction, and it has been shown to work. It generally involves relatively straightforward changes to your diet and lifestyle, which you can make with advice from your GP. You may find some changes harder to make than others.

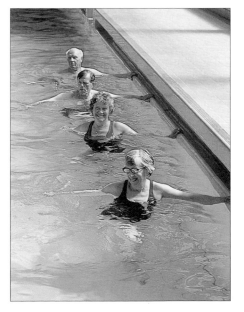

A HEALTHY LIFESTYLE
Leading a healthy lifestyle, including gentle forms of exercise, can help to reduce your blood pressure to normal.

However hard you find it to make the necessary changes, it really is worth making a big effort because, if you are successful, your blood pressure may return to normal without the need for drug treatment. There are several ways in which you can help yourself and really make a difference.

REDUCING SALT INTAKE

Your GP is likely to advise you to reduce the amount of salt you consume. In the UK, the average salt intake in men is 10 grams per day and in women it is about six to seven grams per day. However, a

Amount of Salt Contained in a Selection of Foods

CATEGORY OF FOOD	SALT (G) PER 100 G	CATEGORY OF FOOD	SALT (G) PER 100 G
BREAKFAST CEREALS	0.4–0.9	BEEFBURGERS	0.3–0.6
WHOLEMEAL BREAD	0.4–0.7	BACON	0.8–1.4
SALTED SNACKS	0.5–1.0	TINNED VEGETABLES	0.3–0.7
SAUSAGES	0.8–1.2	FRESH FRUIT	0.1–0.2

very large number of people consume about half this amount, and they have lower blood pressures. Only about one gram of the daily salt intake is added to food when it is on the table or during cooking. The rest comes mostly in processed foods, including burgers, meat pies, sausages, salted snacks, tinned foods (such as vegetables), breakfast cereals and bread.

You can cut your intake by never adding salt to your food at the table or when cooking. Try to make more use of fresh meat and fresh fruit and vegetables, and only eat processed foods as the exception rather than the rule. All herbs and spices are salt free and can be used to flavour foods in place of salt when cooking.

GETTING USED TO LESS SALT

Adjusting to a low-salt diet can be a little difficult at first but you will probably find that, if you can consistently keep your salt intake down, then after about a month or so you actually prefer your food with less salt. If you were then to go back to your old eating habits, you would find that your food tasted too salty and that you have become 'converted'. It is much the same process as happens to people who stop adding large quantities of sugar to their tea or coffee. Once they get used to drinking unsweetened tea or coffee, they often find that adding even a tiny amount of sugar makes it taste so repulsive that they would rather drink water. The same thing can happen when changing from a high-salt to a low-salt diet.

Sadly, the food industry has only responded to the salt/blood pressure problem in a limited manner. Salt was once a useful preservative, but modern food technology and refrigeration mean that the salt content of processed foods can be reduced. Unfortunately, many people have now become 'hooked' on salty foods. There has been some irresponsible propaganda by some representatives of the food industry in which they have suggested that there is no relationship between salt and blood pressure, and that all the experts who have done research in this field are wrong. Experts do not necessarily advocate a drastic reduction in salt intake; they advocate bringing it down to the same level as that in the diets of a great many people who tend to prefer good-quality food without preservatives or additives.

There is some evidence that the lower blood pressures in people in senior positions in executive and managerial jobs are related to their lower salt intake, as well as to the fact that fewer of them are overweight.

SALT SUBSTITUTES

There are several salt substitutes now available from chemist shops. These contain less sodium chloride and more potassium chloride. Although, in an ideal world, no one should need to add crystals of any chemical substance to their food, if you really cannot tolerate food with a low-salt content you can use the salt substitutes instead, provided your kidney function has been shown to be normal. Do not forget, though, that sea salt, rock salt and 'natural' salt are still salt (that is, sodium chloride) and so are not salt substitutes. You need to use salt substitutes with care if you are taking a 'potassium-sparing' drug such as the water pill amiloride, or if your kidneys are not functioning well, because you may have high potassium levels anyway. If in doubt, ask your GP's advice.

WEIGHT CONTROL

As was pointed out on p.37, for every kilogram of weight you lose your blood pressure will fall by about one mmHg.

So, if your blood pressure is only slightly elevated, it may go down to normal if you manage to lose a stone in weight. This is not easy to do, however, unless you have proper advice and strong motivation, and your diet should take account of the need to cut salt intake. Research indicates that, if you are overweight, you are likely to lose more if you are referred to a dietitian than if you are simply told to lose weight by your doctor. You also have a better chance of reaching your target weight if you increase the amount of exercise you take and cut down the alcohol you drink.

SENSIBLE DRINKING

There is good evidence that drinking only moderate amounts of alcohol lowers blood pressure and you probably do not need to give up alcohol altogether.

The Royal Colleges of Physicians, Psychiatrists and General Practitioners in the UK recommend a maximum intake of 21 units of alcohol per week for men and 14 units for women. One unit is the equivalent of half a pint of beer or a small glass of wine (see p.38). Avoid binge drinking because it can cause strokes. The good news is that having one to two drinks every day may be associated with lower levels of heart disease. However, more than four drinks per day does appear to be associated with

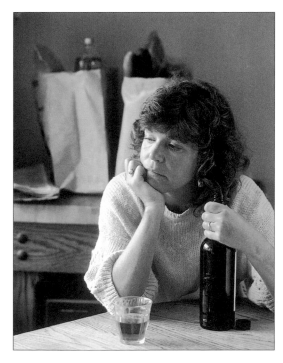

EFFECT OF ALCOHOL
Although a moderate amount of alcohol seems good for the heart, drinking a large amount at any one time may cause strokes.

an increased risk of hypertension and strokes, as well as having damaging effects on the liver, the nervous system and quality of life.

TAKING EXERCISE

Research has proved that there is a clear association between taking more exercise and a fall in blood pressure. The mechanisms are not entirely certain and may in part be related to dietary changes that people often make at the same time as they begin exercising regularly.

If you have hypertension, however, you need to use your common sense when deciding on your exercise programme. For example, an overweight, middle-aged man with severe hypertension who has never taken any exercise would be unwise to take up vigorous exercise that leaves him feeling exhausted. It is much better to opt for a graded programme of gradually increasing exercise. Start by using stairs rather than a lift or escalator when-ever you have to climb only two or three flights, and try walking to a more distant car park or bus stop on the way to and from work or the shops. Any form of sport is fine provided you do not exhaust yourself, but you need to put in sufficient effort to cause a small rise in your pulse rate and make you feel that you are sweating a bit.

POTASSIUM SUPPLEMENTS

Although there is evidence that increasing the amount of potassium in the diet lowers your blood pressure, you should not take supplements in the form of potassium salts or tablets. Instead, you should increase the amount of potassium in your diet by eating more fresh fruit and vegetables, and cut your salt intake from processed foods at the same time.

STRESS COUNSELLING

As explained on p.38, there is little evidence that chronic stress causes high blood pressure. However, there are many people with hypertension who are immensely stressed for a multitude of reasons, as a result of personal problems, anxieties at work or the development of anxiety states for which no obvious cause can be found. If this applies to you, stress counselling and, in extreme cases, psychiatric treatment may help to reduce your stress, and your blood pressure may come down at the same time. Otherwise, there is no reason to believe that most people with hypertension will derive any benefit from stress counselling, relaxation therapies, yoga, biofeedback or other related techniques. What you may find is that, after stress counselling, you are more able to relax when you see your doctor, but this type of treatment for stress does not appear to affect the continuous 24-hour home blood pressure readings that are obtained by using electronic blood pressure monitors. This is a controversial area, but the current view is that the role of stress counselling and the like in the management of hypertension has, to date, been over- rather than understated.

KEY POINTS

- Reducing the amount of salt that you eat will lower your blood pressure.
- Correction of obesity also lowers blood pressure.
- Alcohol consumption should be moderate.
- Exercise can help to lower your blood pressure.

Drug treatment

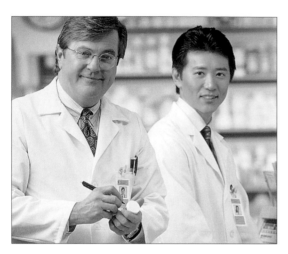

Until the 1950s, there was almost nothing that doctors could do to reduce blood pressure. People with severe hypertension became unwell with strokes, heart and kidney failure, and their doctors could only stand hopelessly by, unable to help.

PRESCRIPTION DRUGS
There are now many anti-hypertensive drugs available on prescription. Over the years, these drugs have been shown to reduce the incidence of heart attacks and strokes.

DRUG DEVELOPMENT

During the late 1950s and early 1960s, antihypertensive drugs became available that did lower blood pressure and did save lives. Many of these early drugs, which are no longer used, were, however, associated with severe side-effects and their use was only justified in patients with a very poor outlook.

During the 1970s, drugs with fewer and less dramatic side-effects became available, and these could therefore be given to people with milder hypertension who were at a lower cardiovascular risk. A large number of well-conducted trials were performed in which active treatment was compared with dummy tablets. All of these trials were discontinued the moment it could be shown that people taking the active treatment developed fewer heart attacks and strokes. Pooling the results of all these trials, we now know that antihypertensive drug therapy for all grades of hypertension brings about a 35–40 per cent reduction of strokes and a 20–25 per cent reduction in coronary heart disease.

People with hypertension may, of course, develop heart attacks as a result of other factors, for example cigarette smoking or having high blood cholesterol levels. It is now, however, true to say that the complications of hypertension should be avoidable if blood pressure can be controlled.

The development of antihypertensive drugs with minimal side-effects and their immense benefits in terms of prevention of heart attacks and strokes has been one of the biggest advances in medical care since World War II. It is at least comparable with the revolution that was achieved with the development of effective antibiotics.

Blood pressure-lowering drugs have also been shown to be effective in reducing or preventing kidney damage in people with diabetes with or without concurrent hypertension, and more recently some drugs have been shown to prevent damage to the retinas of people with diabetes. Furthermore, treatment with certain anti-hypertensive agents can reduce the likelihood of people who have had heart attacks having a second one or developing heart failure.

The publication, in 1997, of a major European study of the treatment of isolated systolic hypertension marks the end of an era. It has left no more room for doubt that anybody with hypertension should be left without treat-ment for more than a few weeks. Everyone whose blood pressure consistently exceeds 160/90 mmHg should take antihypertensive drugs, whatever their age. The only

Drugs Used in the Treatment of Hypertension

The main drugs used in the treatment of hypertension fall into seven main categories, and these are listed below. For more information about each group of drugs, see pp.67–75.

THIAZIDE DIURETICS	bendrofluazide, chlorothiazide, chlorthalidone, cyclopenthiazide, hydrochlorothiazide, indapamide, mefruside, metolazone, polythiazide, xipamide
BETA-BLOCKERS	celiprolol hydrochloride, esmolol hydrochloride, labetalol hydrochloride, metoprolol tartrate, nadolol, oxprenolol hydrochloride, pindolol, sotalol hydrochloride, timolol maleate
CALCIUM CHANNEL BLOCKERS	amlodipine besylate, diltiazem hydrochloride, felodipine, isradipine, lacidipine, lercanidipine hydrochloride, nicardipine hydrochloride, nifedipine, nisoldipine, verapamil hydrochloride
ACE INHIBITORS	captopril, cilazapril, enalapril maleate, fosinopril, lisinopril, moexipril hydrochloride, perindopril, quinapril, ramipril, trandolapril
ALPHA-BLOCKERS	doxazosin, phenoxybenzamine hydrochloride, indoramin, phentolamine mesylate, prazosin, terazosin
CENTRALLY ACTING DRUGS	clonidine hydrochloride, methyldopa, moxonidine
ANGIOTENSIN RECEPTOR ANTAGONISTS	candesartan cilexetil, irbesartan, losartan potassium, valsartan

unanswered question that remains is whether people over the age of 80 benefit from such treatment, and it may be that, in their case, the threshold for beginning therapy should be a little higher than 160/90 mmHg. More information will become available in the near future.

Antihypertensive drug treatment is particularly effective in people aged 60–80 years who, if not given medication of this kind, face a high risk of having a stroke. Older people often worry that they may suffer a stroke, but they can be reassured that drug treatment can largely prevent this happening, which is an excellent reason to keep taking the tablets as prescribed.

CONTROLLING BLOOD PRESSURE

All drugs that lower blood pressure are roughly equally effective. They drop the systolic pressure by about 10–15 mmHg and the diastolic pressure by 6–8 mmHg. Different people respond to the drugs in different ways: for example, older people respond better to some drugs than to others, as do people of Afro-Caribbean origin.

It is worth bearing in mind that much the same falls in blood pressure levels as can be achieved by any single antihypertensive drug can be achieved by someone who sticks rigorously to advice on restricting salt intake, losing weight and drinking only moderate amounts of alcohol. If you are on drug therapy, you should also remember that the effect of some drugs is greater if you reduce your salt consumption while taking them, so it is worth making the necessary effort to cut down your salt intake.

One tablet a day will be enough to control blood pressure for around half the people who are on anti-hypertensive drug therapy. Most of the rest require double therapy with two different drugs, and about 10 per cent of people require triple therapy (that is, three different drugs) to control their blood pressure. Fortunately, even if you need triple therapy, this only means taking three tablets daily. Almost all these can be taken together, either in the morning or in the evening. The older types of drugs, which had to be taken two or three times daily, are now regarded as obsolete. This is obviously good news because the more tablets you have to take every day, the more likely you are to forget to take them sometimes.

If you are one of the small minority of people whose blood pressure proves very difficult to control, you will probably be referred to a specialist, and there are a few people whose blood pressure is almost impossible to control. This is probably because they did not begin taking antihypertensive treatment until a late stage of the disease process, so that the structural changes to the small arterioles are so far advanced that the drugs do not work very well. However, even in this situation, reducing blood pressure does prevent heart attacks and strokes.

It must be stressed, however, that most people who have hypertension have only mildly raised blood pressure that is fairly easily controlled and, if you are in this category, you can be cared for perfectly well by your GP and the practice nurse.

WHO WILL HELP YOU?
If you have only mildly raised blood pressure, your GP will be able to prescibe a drug regime to control your condition.

LONG-TERM TREATMENT

Many people have the mistaken idea that they will need to take drugs to lower their blood pressure only for a short while, rather like taking a short course of antibiotics, and then they can forget the whole thing. This is an extremely dangerous misunderstanding and, if you give up taking the tablets, your risk of a heart attack or a stroke will be greatly increased.

With very few exceptions, antihypertensive treatment needs to be taken for the rest of your life. As you get older, the risk of a stroke increases, and so the benefit of treatment is correspondingly greater. If you stop taking the drugs and your blood pressure stays down, it is necessary to question whether you ever really had hypertension, or whether your treatment was in fact started on the basis of a single raised blood pressure reading taken when you were under stress, just because you were having your blood pressure measured in an unfamiliar environment. In reality, the chances of anyone with genuine hypertension being able to stop antihypertensive tablets are small.

However, if your hypertension was only mild in the first place, and if you needed no more than one tablet a day to control it, then, if you change to a low-salt diet, lose weight, cut down on alcohol and take more exercise, you may be able to come off drug treatment. Even so, about half the people who do manage to do this will need to re-start therapy at some stage. If your doctor does agree that you should stop treatment, he or she will need to see you regularly for check-ups, at first monthly and thereafter three-monthly. It is very likely that your blood pressure will eventually go up again and you will need to go back on the tablets.

Anyone who needs double therapy (two different drugs) to control their blood pressure is extremely unlikely ever to be able to come off therapy altogether. There is, however, some evidence that people whose blood pressure was initially difficult to control, and who therefore needed triple or quadruple therapy, may develop easier blood pressure control as the years go by and so be able to manage on fewer drugs.

Like many people who have been prescribed anti-hypertensive drugs, you may be tempted to stop taking them or actually do so without going back to your doctor. It is all too easy to convince yourself that you do not really need them because you are feeling well and have no symptoms. The chances are that, if you do this, you may one day end up in the accident and emergency department of your local hospital because you have developed one of the complications of hypertension, such as a heart attack or a stroke. Alternatively, you may eventually go back to your doctor with very high blood pressure that is extremely difficult to control, so you then need to take three, four or even five drugs. You can avoid this happening to you if you continue to take the treatment that has been prescribed and attend your doctor's surgery regularly for check-ups.

Following Up Your Treatment

Once your hypertension has been assessed by your doctor and has been brought under control by treatment, you will probably need to have your blood pressure checked only about four times a year.

It is important to go back for such checks to make sure that your blood pressure is under control and, increasingly, your appointments are likely to be with a specially trained practice nurse rather than the doctor.

From time to time, you may need to have other tests besides blood pressure measurement – such as blood tests to check your kidney function or, occasionally, an ECG. Your cholesterol levels should also be monitored because high blood cholesterol, like high blood pressure, is an important risk factor for heart disease and cholesterol-lowering treatment also saves lives.

ANTIHYPERTENSIVE DRUGS

There is now a wide choice of blood pressure-lowering drugs. This means that your doctor is able to tailor the treatment to suit your individual needs. It is important for you to know the names of the drugs that you are taking, how they work and their possible side-effects. With improvements in drug development, it is becoming increasingly possible to minimise side-effects or even avoid them altogether.

The next section of this book describes the currently available drugs. You need to bear in mind that there are usually many different drugs within each of the classes described here and there are minor individual variations between them.

THIAZIDE DIURETICS

These drugs work by opening up blood vessels, which results in a fall in blood pressure, and by helping the kidneys to get rid of salt and water in the urine, which slightly reduces the volume of circulating blood, thus taking some pressure out of the system.

This group of drugs was introduced in the 1950s and they remain the mainstay of treatment for hypertension,

Thiazide Diuretics

- Bendrofluazide
- Chlorothiazide
- Chlorthalidone
- Cyclopenthiazide
- Hydrochlorothiazide
- Indapamide
- Mefruside
- Metolazone
- Polythiazide
- Xipamide

particularly in older people. They are sometimes referred to as 'water tablets' because they slightly increase the production of urine. However, they also tend to relax the medium-sized blood vessels called arterioles, and this helps to explain why they lower blood pressure.

In the early days, thiazide diuretics were used in very high doses. However, it has now become apparent that it is better to take the smallest amount possible while still achieving the desired effect. Higher doses do not work better at lowering blood pressure but do increase the risk of side-effects, such as triggering gout or diabetes. In high doses, thiazide diuretics lower the potassium in the blood and increase the amount of cholesterol or lipids, but such problems are far less prominent now that they are prescribed in sensible low doses.

Among sexually active men, high doses of this type of drug were shown to be associated with impotence. This again has been shown to be much less of a problem now that low doses are used, but even so they are not usually prescribed for sexually active men.

Many of the reported benefits of blood pressure reduction in the various randomised controlled trials described earlier were achieved with this type of drug. They work well for older people and those of Afro-Caribbean origin, and they have almost no noticeable side-effects. They may cause changes in blood chemistry, but these can be minimised if low doses are used.

Some of the thiazide diuretics have a small amount of potassium chloride added to their formulation with the aim of preventing the development of low levels of potassium. In fact, the amount of potassium in the tablets is so small that such combined preparations are no longer recommended. Thiazide diuretics in low dose do not cause a fall in potassium of any great significance, but if this should happen you should be prescribed a different class of drug instead.

BETA-BLOCKERS

These drugs work by blocking the action of noradrenaline that, together with another chemical called adrenaline, prepares the body for emergency situations – the so-called 'flight or fight' response. These powerful chemicals open some blood vessels and narrow others, controlling blood flow to vital organs such as the heart. They also speed up the heart, make it pump more forcibly and push up blood pressure as a result. Beta-blockers stop all this happening and so slow the heart, lessen the force of its contractions and lower blood pressure. However, they also narrow the airways in the lungs, so you cannot take them if you have asthma. And, because they lessen the force of the heart's contraction, they may not be suitable if your heart is not pumping well anyway, for example if you have heart failure.

Beta-blockers were introduced in the 1960s and people found them much easier to take than many of the earlier drugs. They were a mainstay of treatment but, in the 1990s, their use is declining. Some people get on fine with them and experience no side-effects, but on a long-term basis they may subtly reduce your ability to exercise and slightly reduce your energy level as they make your heart pump less forcibly and more slowly. In addition, they may cause cold hands and feet because they reduce the output from the heart. Some, such as propranolol, also

Beta-blockers

- Celiprolol hydrochloride
- Esmolol hydrochloride
- Labetalol hydrochloride
- Metoprolol tartrate
- Nadolol
- Oxprenolol hydrochloride
- Pindolol
- Sotalol hydrochloride
- Timolol maleate

cross into the brain and can cause vivid dreams and sleep disturbance. This is less of a problem with the more modern drugs in this class when used in low doses.

They may not work as well for you if you are of Afro-Caribbean origin, so you are more likely to be prescribed a different type of drug. The same is true of older people.

CALCIUM CHANNEL BLOCKERS

Calcium channel blockers (also known as calcium antagonists) work by blocking the action of calcium in the smooth muscle of the wall of the arterioles. It is thought that constriction of the smooth muscle, caused in part by calcium, narrows these blood vessels, which causes hypertension to develop. Blocking the action of calcium opens up the blood vessels and results in a fall in blood pressure.

The problem is that all arterioles open up, including the ones in the brain, which can lead to headaches; ones in the face, which can cause flushing; and ones in the legs, which can result in ankle swelling; but the newer, longer-acting formulations produce far fewer side-effects of this kind. Nifedipine is now prescribed in this long-acting formulation and, although amlodipine and lacidipine cause few problems, high doses do cause ankle swelling. This is not due to heart failure and is not sinister; however, some women in particular may find it unacceptable.

Another calcium channel blocker (verapamil) can cause constipation and may also be hazardous in certain forms of heart disease.

During 1995, anxieties were expressed about the safety of calcium channel blockers, but these

Calcium Channel Blockers

- Amlodipine besylate
- Diltiazem hydrochloride
- Felodipine
- Isradipine
- Lacidipine
- Lercanidipine hydrochloride
- Nicardipine hydrochloride
- Nifedipine
- Nisoldipine
- Verapamil hydrochloride

anxieties were allayed by the publication of a major trial in 1997, which showed that these drugs prevent heart attacks and strokes and are not associated with an excess of other problems. They are particularly effective in older people and those of Afro-Caribbean origin.

ACE INHIBITORS

ACE (angiotensin-converting enzyme) inhibitors work by preventing the activation of the hormone angiotensin II from its two precursors, renin and angiotensin I. Because angiotensin II constricts blood vessels, ACE inhibitors effectively open up the blood vessels, resulting in a lowering of blood pressure.

This class of drug represents an important breakthrough in the management of hypertension. Not only do these drugs lower blood pressure, they also protect the kidneys of people with diabetes and hypertension. More recently, they have been shown also to delay the onset of retinal damage, which can impair the vision of people with diabetes. They are also prescribed for some people who have recovered from a heart attack.

ACE inhibitors are remarkably safe but, if you are already on water pills (diuretics), you need to be monitored closely by your doctor when you first start taking them because the first dose can cause a sudden fall in blood pressure. Newer ACE inhibitors are less prone to do this, but you may be advised to stop diuretics for a day or so before starting treatment with an ACE inhibitor. ACE inhibitors are very effective in the treatment of congestive heart failure, whether or not blood pressure is raised.

ACE Inhibitors

- Captopril
- Cilazapril
- Enalapril maleate
- Fosinopril
- Lisinopril
- Moexipril hydrochloride
- Perindopril
- Quinapril
- Ramipril
- Trandolapril

Around one in 1,000 people of Afro-Caribbean origin, and one in 4,000 white people, experience an acute allergic response to this type of drug – their tongue and lips swell and their upper airways become constricted. This happens rarely but is not always recognised for what it is. The only other important side-effect of this class of drugs is that they cause a dry, irritating cough in about 10 per cent of men and 20 per cent of women. This cough has no sinister significance and may not bother you too much, although your partner may complain that your cough keeps him or her awake at night.

ACE inhibitors have no adverse effects on mental function because they do not cross into the brain, unlike the early beta-blockers, and most people get on very well indeed with them. However, these drugs do not work particularly well when given on their own to people of Afro-Caribbean origin and to older people, who may need to take a thiazide diuretic or a calcium channel blocker at the same time.

ALPHA-BLOCKERS

These work by blocking the action of the chemical adrenaline on muscles that make up the walls of blood vessels. Adrenaline makes the blood vessels constrict and pushes up blood pressure. Blocking these receptors makes the blood vessels relax and blood pressure falls. As a result of this, alpha-blockers can also cause dizziness, especially when you stand up suddenly, but, other than that, they have few side-effects.

The early alpha-blockers needed to be given three times a day and caused side-effects of dizziness, light-headedness and a dry mouth. More

Alpha-blockers

- Doxazosin
- Indoramin
- Phenoxybenzamine hydrochloride
- Phentolamine mesylate
- Prazosin
- Terazosin

recently, two alpha-blockers that can be taken once daily have been introduced: doxazosin and terazosin. They are entirely safe but may still cause some dizziness in some individuals.

Alpha-receptor blockers work on other parts of the body as well as blood pressure. They have been shown, in particular, to relax the bladder, and this is useful for elderly men with enlarged prostates who have difficulty passing water. By contrast, they may occasionally cause some stress incontinence among women. This is reversible once the tablets are stopped.

CENTRALLY ACTING DRUGS

These work by acting on the part of the brain that controls blood pressure. These drugs are very rarely used now. Although they are entirely safe, they do tend to cause tiredness, lethargy and even depression, particularly in high doses.

> ## Centrally Acting Drugs
>
> - Clonidine hydrochloride
> - Methyldopa
> - Moxonidine

Newer drugs, which work in different ways, have fewer side-effects and are equally safe, so methyldopa is now usually used only when other drugs have been found to be ineffective in reducing blood pressure. It is still prescribed for pregnant women, for whom it is known to be entirely safe. For very good reasons, doctors tend to prescribe drugs in pregnancy only if they have been available for a great many years. This is simply because the world experience is such that they can be confident that there will be no adverse effects on the developing baby. There is good evidence that methyldopa is safe in pregnancy. If you are given it while pregnant, however, you will probably change to another type of drug after the birth if your blood pressure still requires treatment.

ANGIOTENSIN RECEPTOR ANTAGONISTS

These work in a similar way to ACE inhibitors, but by blocking the angiotensin II receptors rather than by blocking the activation of angiotensin II. For this reason, they have a more specific effect on blood pressure and do not cause troublesome side-effects such as a cough.

This new class of drug was introduced in 1995 and rapidly became popular because these drugs appear to have fewer side-effects than all the other classes of drugs. They lower blood pressure effectively and have been shown to be remarkably safe. As yet there are no long-term studies of their use and a great many trials are currently underway.

Angiotensin receptor antagonists share a great many of the actions of the ACE inhibitors and some of the actions of the beta-blockers. For this reason, they might be expected to work less well for older people and those of Afro-Caribbean origin, but we do not yet know for sure whether this is actually the case. They may, as with the ACE inhibitors, also be particularly beneficial for people with kidney disease and heart disease, but new information is constantly becoming available.

COMBINATION THERAPIES

As explained on p.63, about half of those people with hypertension need to take more than one drug to control it, but usually this will only mean taking a maximum of four tablets a day, sometimes fewer. Certain combinations of drugs are more effective than others. Although there are many exceptions, in general the beta-blockers and ACE inhibitors are best given with either thiazide diuretics or calcium channel blockers. There is often not

Angiotensin Receptor Antagonists

- Candesartan cilexetil
- Irbesartan
- Losartan potassium
- Valsartan

much to be gained by combining a beta-blocker with an ACE inhibitor or combining a thiazide diuretic with a calcium channel blocker. If you are one of the minority of people who needs three drugs to control your blood pressure, then there are probably no important drug interactions. It is considered best to use two or more blood pressure-lowering drugs in lower doses rather than any one drug in a high dose. All drugs can be taken together once daily so even quadruple therapy requires only four pills taken together. To help patients who require combination therapies, there are several blood pressure-lowering tablets that contain two different drugs that work well together (for example, Tenoret 50, Zestoretic and Cozaar-Comp).

AFRO-CARIBBEAN PEOPLE

Hypertension is very common among people who are of Afro-Caribbean origin. In the USA, it is twice as common as in the white and Hispanic populations. The picture is much the same in the UK, as well as in urban societies

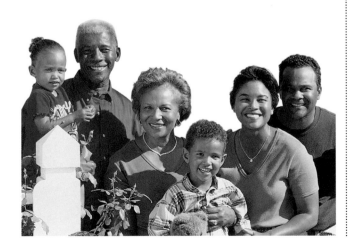

ETHNIC RISKS
There may be a variety of reasons why Afro-Caribbeans are twice as likely to have high blood pressure than white people, but salt intake appears to be a major factor.

in Africa. By sharp contrast, in rural Africa hypertension is relatively uncommon.

There is reasonably good evidence that the increased prevalence of hypertension in the African-origin community in the UK and the USA is related to salt intake. In Africa, with increasing urbanisation, there is a sharp increase in salt intake with a moderate reduction in potassium intake, and both of these effects are contributing to the rise in people's blood pressure. Within the UK and the USA, there is less convincing evidence that people of Afro-Caribbean origin consume more salt than anyone else, although in the USA they tend to have a diet that is low in potassium because they eat less fresh fruit and vegetables. It does appear, however, that people of Afro-Caribbean origin may be more sensitive to a given salt load than those from different racial backgrounds.

Possibly as a result of the increased sensitivity to salt, people of Afro-Caribbean origin who have hypertension have been shown to have lower levels of the hormones renin and angiotensin II in their blood. This is important because, as we have seen, some of the drugs that lower blood pressure do so by blocking the effects of these particular hormones. It will come as no surprise therefore that these drugs are less effective in people who have low renin and angiotensin levels in the first place. So, although beta-blockers, ACE inhibitors and probably angiotensin receptor antagonists may not work well for you if you are of Afro-Caribbean origin, drugs that work in a different way, such as thiazide diuretics, calcium channel blockers, alpha-blockers and possibly centrally acting drugs, offer effective alternatives.

Another important factor is that diabetes is three times more common in Afro-Caribbean people in the UK compared with white people, and diabetes and hypertension commonly occur together. If you have both, your risk of developing cardiovascular disease is higher. This means that your doctor is likely to want you to start on antihypertensive drugs even though your blood pressure may be only slightly raised. In fact, the current view is that everyone, from whatever ethnic background, who has both diabetes and hypertension should receive this type of treatment if their blood pressure consistently exceeds 140/90 mmHg.

In the UK, and to a lesser extent in the USA, coronary heart disease (that is, heart attacks and angina) is relatively less common in people of Afro-Caribbean origin who have high blood pressure. On the other hand, strokes and kidney failure are more common among these people. The reasons for these ethnic differences are not entirely certain, but, from a practical point of view, if you do belong to the Afro-Caribbean community, you need to take on board the importance of restricting your salt intake, having your blood pressure measured regularly and being prepared to start (and keep taking) drug treatment if your blood pressure is consistently high.

ASIANS AND HYPERTENSION
South-east Asians living in the UK commonly develop high blood pressure, due in part to eating a high-fat Western diet.

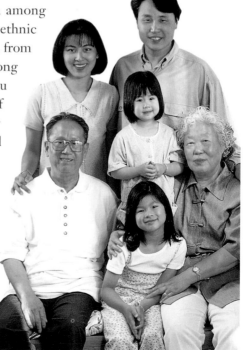

ASIAN PEOPLE

People of south Asian origin who live in the UK are more prone to develop hypertension than their white neighbours. This is thought to be probably related to a greater tendency to be overweight and to a higher frequency of developing diabetes. The rates of coronary heart disease (angina and heart attacks) in Asian communities in the UK are very high, possibly in part because some of these individuals consume large amounts of fatty foods.

As in the Afro-Caribbean community, however, the ethnic difference in the rates of disease remains partly unexplained. People from an Asian background do not seem, on the basis of current evidence, to respond any differently from white people to the various classes of antihypertensive drugs.

OTHER ETHNIC GROUPS

At present, we know relatively little about hypertension and the risks associated with it as regards to other ethnic groups in the UK. Some people of Chinese origin consume large amounts of salt in their food, and this may explain the high incidence of strokes in both China and Japan. There is almost no information on this topic from the UK. Having said that, the advice given earlier about cutting down salt is worth following, whatever your ethnic background. There is no evidence that any of the Oriental herbs or spices are harmful in any way. Be careful, however, about Oriental herbal remedies that are imported from China. Some are very toxic and there is no quality control of their contents. Lifestyle advice is the

EATING SENSIBLY
Even if you do not belong to a high risk ethnic group, it is worth following a low-fat, low-salt, fruit- and vegetable-rich diet.

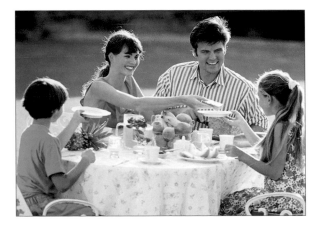

same for everyone: a high-fat, high-salt diet is bad for your cardiovascular health whereas a low-fat, low-salt, high fruit and vegetable diet is beneficial and will help to protect you against ill health in general and cardiovascular disease in particular. Whatever ethnic group you belong to, you should also avoid drinking excessive amounts of alcohol and make a point of taking more exercise.

KEY POINTS

- There is a wide choice of antihypertensive drugs.
- All antihypertensive drugs are roughly equally effective.
- About half of all people who are hypertensive need two or more drugs to control their blood pressure.
- The more modern drugs have fewer side-effects.

Special cases

Some medical conditions and groups of people require special consideration with regard to high blood pressure. This is to ensure that the correct antihypertensive medication and preventative treatment can be prescribed.

Those who require special attention include people suffering from particular illnesses or taking certain kinds of drugs, children, the elderly and pregnant women.

PREGNANCY

Your blood pressure usually stays the same or falls a little while you are pregnant. Some women actually find out that it is high during pregnancy, but this is because it has been that way for some time and they have not had it checked before. In this situation, it is purely coincidental and not really related to pregnancy; it just happens to be detected while you are pregnant.

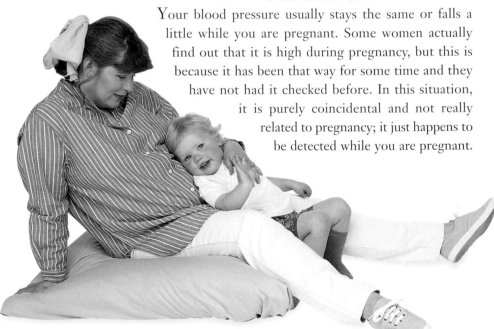

Its management is the same as for anyone else who is diagnosed with hypertension, although the choice of drugs may well be different.

MILDLY RAISED BLOOD PRESSURE

About 25 per cent of women expecting their first baby develop slightly raised blood pressure in the last three months of pregnancy. If they do not have any kidney damage and no protein appears in the urine on testing, then drug therapy may not be given to bring the pressure down. The significance of mildly raised blood pressure in pregnancy is uncertain, but careful monitoring is crucial.

PRE-ECLAMPSIA

Pre-eclampsia is a different matter and is potentially very serious for you and your baby. It affects about five per cent of women in the second half of their first pregnancies and is defined as a blood pressure of over 160/90 mmHg; a urine test will usually show that you have protein in your urine.

If undetected, pre-eclampsia can progress into a very serious condition called eclampsia, in which the woman has fits and both mother and baby are in danger. Hospital admission and specialised treatment are necessary. The cause of this condition is not yet fully understood or preventable. Pre-eclampsia is less common in second and third pregnancies (if the pregnancy is by the same father).

REGULAR CHECKS

Your blood pressure and urine are checked for signs of pre-eclampsia every time you attend the antenatal clinic. If you have been prescribed antihypertensive drug treatment for the first time while you are pregnant, you will probably be able to come off it once your baby is about two weeks old, but your doctors will want you to come back for regular check-ups. Many women who have had hypertension in their first pregnancy will have no further trouble next time round. It is possible that you may be at greater risk of developing it in later life, and you will need to carry on having your blood pressure checked, perhaps once a year.

SUITABLE DRUGS

In pregnancy, there is a severe limit to the choice of blood pressure-lowering drugs. Methyldopa and labetalol are safe, but atenolol is probably best avoided because it may result in underweight babies. ACE inhibitors should never be used in pregnancy under any circumstances. If high blood pressure is resistant to therapy, then nifedipine may be added, although there is only limited information about its use.

CHEST DISEASE

The most important point is that you cannot take betablocker drugs if you have any form of wheeze, asthma or similar breathing difficulties, but there is no problem as regards other antihypertensive drugs. ACE inhibitors can cause a dry, irritating cough, but this is not usually associated with breathlessness. The cough will disappear once you stop taking the tablets and there are plenty of alternative treatments.

ANGINA

If you suffer from angina, you will need detailed assessment, including blood tests to measure your cholesterol levels and, if they prove necessary, cholesterol-reducing drugs. Beta-blocker drugs may be particularly helpful at reducing the frequency of angina attacks, but you will need to be carefully monitored by your doctor while taking these drugs.

■ HEART ATTACK ■

After a heart attack you may benefit from taking a lipid-lowering drug, such as simvastatin, to lower your cholesterol levels to mini-mise the risk of a further heart attack. ACE inhibitors and beta-blockers may have additional advantages from your point of view because, as well as controlling your blood pressure, they make the heart work less hard and help to protect the heart muscle from further damage. Your doctor will usually recommend that you take low-dose aspirin every day.

TAKING A BLOOD SAMPLE
If you suffer from angina, your blood will probably be tested to assess cholesterol levels. If these are high, cholesterol-lowering drugs may be prescribed.

AFTER A STROKE

If you have had the misfortune to have a stroke, lowering your blood pressure rapidly could be harmful but, on a longer-term basis, keeping your blood pressure under careful control may reduce the risk of you suffering a recurrence.

The choice of drug treatment will be up to your doctor, and the fact that you have had a stroke does not mean that you cannot take some drugs or that others would be spe-cially appropriate. If tests show your stroke was caused by a cerebral thrombosis (a blood clot in the brain), as opposed to a cerebral haemorrhage (bleeding in the brain), then you will be prescribed aspirin in a low dose.

DEPRESSION

If you have a tendency to be depressed or worried about your hypertension, it is worth remembering that anti-hypertensive drug therapy has been the great medical success story of the last 50 years because it brings about a massive reduction in heart attack and strokes.

The older beta-blockers, such as propranolol, and the centrally acting drug methyldopa, may not be suitable for you because they can be associated with depression, lethargy and tiredness, so if you have a tendency towards depression these drugs are best avoided. The thiazide diuretics and the newer classes of antihypertensive drugs appear to have no effects on mood.

If your depression is being treated with lithium therapy, you should not take thiazide diuretics for hypertension because your blood lithium levels may then rise to potentially hazardous levels.

THE CONTRACEPTIVE PILL

Most oral contraceptives cause a tiny and unimportant rise in blood pressure. The diastolic blood pressure rises to more than 90 mmHg in about five per cent of women - usually those who are older, overweight and with a past history of slightly raised blood pressure readings. Only in rare circumstances can the contraceptive pill alone cause severe hypertension with a level that requires treatment.

There is evidence that the newer, low-dose, combined oral preparations and the progesterone-only pills cause a smaller rise in blood pressure than the older, high-dose, combined preparations. You may be able to take the combined oral contraceptive pill even if you have hypertension, provided you are carefully monitored by your doctor. It is particularly important to avoid becoming overweight. Many of the complications that may result from taking oral contraceptive pills affect older women who are also cigarette smokers.

HRT

The amount of oestrogen in hormone replacement therapy (HRT) is much smaller than that in the oral contraceptive pill. In the past, doctors have been somewhat cautious about prescribing HRT for women with hypertension, but recent surveys suggest this is quite safe provided you are carefully monitored by your doctor. Hypertension on its own is not a reason for not taking HRT, but you do have to avoid putting on a lot of weight, which can sometimes happen with this treatment. There is no evidence that HRT in any way interferes with antihypertensive drugs.

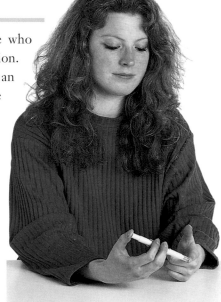

BEING VIGILANT
In addition to checking blood glucose levels regularly, as this girl is doing, diabetics should also have their blood pressure taken at regular intervals. The combination of hypertension and diabetes greatly increases the risk of eye and kidney damage and heart disease.

DIABETES

Hypertension is more common in people who have diabetes than in the rest of the population. If you have both conditions, you have an increased risk of developing damage to the eyes and the kidneys, as well as coronary heart disease and stroke.

Apart from maintaining good blood glucose control, you need to make an effort to avoid becoming overweight, your cholesterol levels need to be checked and treated if raised and your blood pressure must be kept under very strict control indeed. There is evidence that one class of drugs, the ACE inhibitors, is better than other drugs at preventing kidney and eye damage in type 1 diabetes (that is, diabetes needing treatment by insulin injection).

In 1998, a very important study was published that showed that lowering the blood pressure to below 140/85 mmHg in people with type 2 diabetes was extremely beneficial. So, although the threshold for starting drug treatment is 160/90 mmHg for people who do not have diabetes, for those who do the threshold should be 130–140/85 mmHg.

CHILDREN

Severely raised blood pressure in children is rare and is usually associated with significant kidney conditions; such children should be seen in specialist children's hospitals. Overweight children and those children with a strong family history of hypertension may have slightly raised blood pressure.

OVERWEIGHT CHILDREN
Obese children, especially those with high blood pressure in their families, have a tendency to develop hypertension.

If you have hypertension, you should be aware that your children are at risk of developing this condition too. Make sure that your childrens' diet is as low in salt as possible and, in particular, do not let them eat too many crisps or other salted snacks or too many convenience foods such as burgers. It is also important not to let them get fat.

Very rarely, high blood pressure can be the result of autosomal dominant polycystic kidney disease. This is usually diagnosed in adult life, but a parent with the condition needs to know that 50 per cent of his or her children are likely to have this condition. If you have autosomal dominant polycystic kidney disease, you should arrange for your children to be screened for this condition.

ELDERLY PEOPLE

Some years ago, elderly people were seen as a separate subgroup who needed to be treated differently from younger people, but this view is now known to be spurious. As you get older, your blood pressures rises and the risk of heart attack and strokes becomes correspondingly greater. Recent treatment trials have shown that antihypertensive treatment is particularly effective in older people and a great many heart attacks and strokes can be prevented. Older people do have a higher frequency of other conditions, including diabetes and arthritis and, if you have a condition such as these, you may require different antihypertensive drugs.

Otherwise, treatment for hypertension is the same, whatever your age. If your blood pressure is persistently greater than 160/90 mmHg, even after you have followed the advice on lifestyle changes outlined on pp.53–59, you will need to start taking antihypertensive drugs. There is a trend for the thiazide diuretics and the calcium channel blockers to be more effective, and the ACE inhibitors and the beta-blockers less effective, in older patients. Sometimes, you may need to take two different drugs in low dose rather than any one drug in high dose. You can be reassured that controlling your blood pressure with drugs is particularly effective at preventing strokes. There is no reason why you should not lead a normal, active life while making sure that you follow a healthy diet that does not contain too much salt, but contains adequate amounts of potassium-rich fruit and vegetables.

KEY POINTS

- Pregnant women need careful blood pressure assessment, and drug treatment is occasionally necessary.

- Concomitant heart disease, chest disease and diabetes influence choice of blood pressure-lowering drugs.

- Blood pressure in people aged over 65 is managed in exactly the same way as in younger people, and this definitely prevents heart attacks and strokes.

Questions and answers

What is hypertension?

Hypertension is simply the state of having a blood pressure that is rather higher than average. If sustained, it can increase the risk of having a heart attack or a stroke.

Can anything be done about it?

Yes, lowering blood pressure definitely prevents heart attacks and strokes.

How can I find out whether I have hypertension?

The only way to find out whether you have high blood pressure is to have it measured by your doctor or practice nurse. I am afraid that there is no association between high blood pressure and any specific symptoms, including headache. All adults should have a routine blood pressure check.

How can I get my blood pressure down?

You can help to reduce your blood pressure by adopting a low-salt diet with plenty of fresh fruit and vegetables. In addition, you should try to avoid becoming overweight and consume only moderate amounts of alcohol.

What happens if this is not effective?

If your blood pressure cannot be lowered by non-drug therapies alone, then drug therapy is quite often necessary. There is, however, a wide choice of blood pressure-lowering drugs and it can almost be guaranteed that that you will have no side-effects.

The most important thing to remember is that, if your blood pressure is controlled, your risk of having a heart attack or a stroke is greatly reduced.

Will I be able to stop my treatment?

You should only discontinue anti-hypertensive drugs under medical supervision with careful follow-up. Almost all patients need to take their drugs indefinitely for the rest of their lives. Even if you are able to stop the therapy, you will still have to be seen at least every few months for re-checking.

What is the cause of high blood pressure?

High blood pressure appears to result from the interplay of genetic (inherited) factors and lifestyle factors. There is a tendency in all Western societies to consume large quantities of salt in food. In addition, being overweight or obese can cause high blood pressure, as can excess alcohol consumption. In a very small minority of people, we can find underlying kidney diseases that are the cause of high blood pressure.

However, at the end of the day we do not know all of the answers to this question.

Will high blood pressure or its treatment affect my quality of life?
Definitely not. Modern drugs are virtually free of side effects. You are encouraged to return to a normal, active, busy and interesting life. Only people with very high blood pressure need to stop work, and even then only briefly.

How common is hypertension?
About seven million British citizens have raised blood pressure. Not all of them need drug treatment, but they all need careful supervision by their GP or practice nurse.

Useful addresses

**British Hypertension Society
Information Service**
Blood Pressure Unit
St George's Hospital Medical School
Cranmer Terrace
London SW17 0RE
Tel: (020) 8725 3412
For leaflets, self-help guidance and advice
on home monitoring devices.

British Heart Foundation
14 Fitzhardinge Street
London W1H 4DH
Tel: (020) 7935 0185
Helpline: 0870 6006566
Website: www.bhf.org.uk

Notes

Index

Acknowledgements

PUBLISHER'S ACKNOWLEDGEMENTS
Dorling Kindersley would like to thank the following for their help
and participation in this project:

Editorial Assistance Alyson McGaw; **Production** Michelle Thomas;
DTP Jason Little; **Consultancy** Dr. Sue Davidson;
Indexing Indexing Specialists, Hove; **Administration** Christopher Gordon.

Illustrations (p.11, p.23) © Gillian Lee, (p.30) © Debbie Maizels

Picture Research Andy Sansom; **Picture Librarian** Charlotte Oster.

PICTURE CREDITS
The publisher would like to thank the following for their kind
permission to reproduce their photographs. Every effort has been made
to trace the copyright holders. Dorling Kindersley apologises for any
unintentional omissions and would be pleased, in any such cases,
to add an acknowledgement in future editions.

Sally and Richard Greenhill p.53; **Science Photo Library** p.20, (Dr. P. Marazzi),
p.40 (Maximillian Stock Ltd.), p.47 (Paul Parker), p.86 (CC Studio); **Telegraph Colour Library** p.7
(Steve Bloom), p.75 (Rob Gage); **Tony Stone Images**, p.10 (Darryl Torckler), p.34, p.48 (Charles
Gupton), p.57 (David Young Wolff), p.60 (Bruce Ayres), p.77 (Jon Riley), p.78 (Peter Correz)